JEWISH ALCOHOLISM
AND
DRUG ADDICTION

JEWISH ALCOHOLISM
AND
DRUG ADDICTION
An Annotated Bibliography

Compiled by
STEVEN L. BERG

Bibliographies and Indexes in Ethnic Studies, Number 5

GREENWOOD PRESS
Westport, Connecticut • London

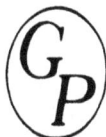

Library of Congress Cataloging-in-Publication Data

Berg, Steven L.
    Jewish alcoholism and drug addiction : an annotated bibliography /
compiled by Steven L. Berg.
        p.   cm. – (Bibliographies and indexes in ethnic studies, ISSN
1046-7882 ; no. 5)
    Includes index.
    ISBN 0-313-27603-X (alk. paper)
    1. Jews—Alcohol use—Bibliography. 2. Jews—Drug use—
Bibliography. 3. Alcoholism—Bibliography. 4. Drug abuse—
Bibliography.   I. Title. II. Series.
    Z7721.B45   1993
    [HV5185]
    016.3629'089924—dc20   93-21634

British Library Cataloguing in Publication Data is available.

Library of Congress Catalog Card Number: 93-21634
ISBN: 0-313-27603-X
ISSN: 1046-7882

First published in 1993

Greenwood Press, 88 Post Road West, Westport, CT 06881
An imprint of Greenwood Publishing Group, Inc.

Printed in the United States of America

∞™

The paper used in this book complies with the
Permanent Paper Standard issued by the National
Information Standards Organization (Z39.48-1984).

10 9 8 7 6 5 4 3 2 1

dedicated to

RICHARD J. KOEHN
VALERIE PRZYWARA

and to the memory of

FRANK SCHEER

Contents

Preface

Funding for *Jewish Alcoholism and Drug Addiction* was originally provided by Guest House, Inc. But I am especially indebted to the following people whose financial support insured the completion of the research: Andrew Stuart, Harvey Ballard, Barbara Harte, Mary Hartshorn, Christopher Berg, and Lorain and Judy Berg. Without them, this book would never have been completed.

Family has always played an important role in my research. In addition to the individuals named above, I have been nourished by other family members and friends: Mike and Janice Berg, Marty Carlson, David Smith, G.C. Landon, Jacque Shoppell, Robert Sanchez, Michael and Crystal Yachcik. There was also my grandmother, Rachel Liberacki, who did not live long enough to see this book in print but helped me celebrate when Greenwood Press offered me the contract.

My nephew, Alex, is too young to remember sitting on his uncle's knee while helping operate the computer, but he was a joyful research companion. Christopher Prell also helped in his own way. Eric Mattlin graciously allowed me to hide away in his home in order to work on the manuscript. Nancy and Mike Meyer helped insure that this research was not lost. LuAnn Beamer served as a research assistant. Don Hallog, Chair of the English Division at Delta College has encouraged me in my teaching.

Members of SALIS (Substance Abuse Librarians and Information Specialists) have been consistently supportive of my research. I especially wish to thank Cathy Weglarz in this regard. Several individuals shared their research with me: Nochem Gringras, Marcia Cohn Spiegel, Ernie Kurtz, Syd Abrams. Charles Bishop, Jr. hosted me in his home so that I could have access to his extensive library. There are also those people who call themselves the Back Porch Group.

It was Richard J. Koehn's foresight that lead to the creation of the "Spiritual Issues Bibliography" which I began to compile in 1987 and from which this book has grown. Dick, rightly, saw no reason why Catholics and Jews could not work together to help the still suffering alcoholics and those who love them. It is only right that this book should be dedicated to him. Valerie Przywara has been a friend in many, many ways. Those who knew Frank Scheer and loved him as I did understand why he shares the dedication with Dick and Valerie.

Introduction

Jewish Alcoholism and Drug Addiction: An Annotated Bibliography is the third publication from a larger project on the relationship between spirituality and recovery from addiction. The first was my dissertation "AA, Spiritual Issues, and the Treatment of Lesbian and Gay Alcoholics" (Berg, 1989a). The second was the anthology *Alcoholism and Pastoral Ministry: Readings on Recovery* (Berg, 1989b). Through cooperation with members of SALIS (Substance Abuse Librarians and Information Specialists) and the Center of Alcohol Studies at Rutgers University, it is my hope that the information compiled as part of these and future publications will continue to serve people interested in quality reference materials on alcoholism/other drug addiction, spirituality, and minority populations.

METHODOLOGY AND SCOPE OF THE BIBLIOGRAPHY

Jewish Alcoholism and Drug Addiction is a comprehensive bibliography. Any reference which mentioned alcoholism and other drug addiction within the Jewish community was included in the text regardless of the quality of the article. For a period of time, the *Journal of Studies on Alcohol* included excellent summaries of current literature. While I found these summaries to be extremely useful in tracking down articles for this bibliography, the summaries themselves are not cited here. Also, books whose only value was that they included an article on the topic are not included. For example, Charles Snyder's (1962) "Culture and Jewish Sobriety" which appeared in *Society, Culture, and Drinking Practices* (Pittman and Snyder, 1962) is included, but Pittman and Snyder's book is not.

This bibliography was primarily researched by tracking back footnotes and bibliographic references and then by investigating the references included in the newly discovered sources. *Addictions in the Jewish Community* (Levy and Blume, 1986) and *Alcoholism and the Jewish Community* (Blaine, 1980) served as the starting point for the research. In addition to the leads from these two books, I identified materials by using a data base search done by the National Clearinghouse on Alcoholism and Drug Addiction, *The Annotated Bibliography of Alcoholics Anonymous, 1939-1989* (Bishop & Pittman, 1989), *The NALGAP [National Association of Lesbian and Gay Alcoholism Professionals] Annotated Bibliography: Alcoholism, Substance Abuse, and Lesbians/Gay Men* (Berg, Finnegan, & McNally, 1987), and the *Index to Jewish Periodicals*. In addition, I am indebted to Marcia Cohn Spiegel, Rabbi Nochem Gringras, Sydney Abrams, and Ernie Kurtz for sharing research materials with me.

The citations in the book follow the general guidelines of the American Psychological Association. The following abbreviations are used throughout: (n.a.) for "no author," (n.d.) for "no date," and (n.p.) for "no publisher."

Annotations are descriptive and not evaluative and focus on the Jewish material included in the citation. Index terms are taken from the article and not from the annotation. As a result, they are more comprehensive than the annotations. Entry numbers refer to bibliographic entries and not to page numbers.

Forcing essays into artificial categories is always problematic because selections frequently fit into more than one category. Emily McNally's (1989) excellent "Lesbian Recovering Alcoholics in Alcoholics Anonymous" is one such reference. Her dissertation, in which two of the eight women studied were Jewish, could easily have fit under the following categories: empirical studies, Jews in AA, women, testimonials and case studies, and lesbian/gay issues. Because McNally's dissertation places an emphasis on lesbianism, I placed it in the lesbian/gay category. However, my own dissertation on "AA, Spiritual Issues, and the Treatment of Lesbian and Gay Alcoholics" (1989a) is found under the category "Jews in AA" because the Jewish material in it focuses on difficulties which some Jews have in AA and not on the lesbian/gay Jewish experience. Because each reference is listed only once, the reader is encouraged to consult the index as well as the chapter headings.

ORGANIZATION OF CHAPTERS AND INDEXES

Chapter 1 includes references to general studies of addiction within the Jewish community. References where there was only a brief mention of alcoholism or other drug addiction are also found in the first chapter.

Chapters 2 and 3 focus on scholarly studies. Empirical studies are found in the second chapter while the third includes those essays which are more theoretical.

Because Judaism is considered both a religion and a culture, many studies have focused on the relationship of Jewish alcoholics and addicts to other religions and cultures. If a study compares the followers of Judaism to other religious traditions, it will be found in chapter 4. If the comparison is to other cultural groups, the reference will be found in chapter 5.

The sixth chapter combines first person stories and case studies of Jewish addicts and alcoholics. First person stories are, of course, told from the individuals point of view. Case studies are written in the third person.

Two organizations which have been significant in helping Jewish alcoholics and other drug addicts are Alcoholics Anonymous (AA) and Jewish Alcoholics, Chemically Dependent Persons, and Significant Others (JACS). References which focus on AA are found in chapter 7 while material relating to JACS is found in chapter 8.

The rabbi has traditionally had an important impact on chemically dependant Jews and their families. The references in

Chapter 9 show how the rabbi can have either a positive or negative impact on the congregation. The fact that rabbis are not immune to addiction is also shown in this chapter.

In chapter 10, the focus is on alcoholism in Israel.

Although Jews are a minority in the United States, I believe it is important to recognize that there are minorities within the Jewish community. Therefore, chapter 11 includes references to women, youth, lesbians, gay men, and blacks.

The final chapter shows how Jewish alcoholics are portrayed in literature.

Because many references can fit in more than one category, it is important for the reader to use the three indexes which are provided: author, title, and subject. The author index includes not only names of the authors whose works are mentioned in the references, but also authors who are mentioned in various citations. As with the authors, titles also include mention of other titles within a work. A reader who uses the subject index to find a reference in the book might be surprised to find no mention of the subject in the citation. This is because the subject index was from the original and not from the annotations which appear in this book. As a result, the index is more complete than the citations.

AVAILABILITY OF MATERIALS

The library which I built to support this project has been donated to the Center of Alcohol Studies at Rutgers University and is being housed there as one of their special collections. Researchers are welcome to use the collection at Rutgers. The library is able to supply photocopies of non-book items for a small fee. Requests for materials should be sent to the Center of Alcohol Studies Libraries, Box 969, Piscataway, NJ 08855-0969. Please be sure to include the author, title, and place of publication when making a request. The citation number from this bibliography would also be helpful.

THEMES IN THE LITERATURE

The major theme in the literature is that Jews have a natural immunity to alcoholism; an immunity that explains the low rate of addiction in the Jewish community. This immunity has been attributed to both cultural and religious factors. Because this idea is so central to Jewish thinking on addiction, even those authors who recognize the myth of Jewish immunity must deal with the issue before they begin to describe educational programs.

The main cultural factor which is attributed to the high rate of sobriety among Jews is that Jews, as an oppressed people, needed to be constantly on guard. Gentiles might be afforded the luxury of getting drunk, but drunkenness and the actions typically associated with that condition could only further the discrimination Jews faced in a hostile world.

The fact that Jews are introduced to alcohol at an early age and typically have strong family ties has also been cited to support the theory of Jewish immunity as has the religious significance of wine in Jewish ritual.

For those people who accept the myth that Jews are immune to drug abuse, the increase in alcoholism and other drug addiction is a result of assimilation. These people argue that as Jews lose their cultural and religious traditions by mainstreaming into Gentile society, they also lose those co-factors which have historically been attributed to their low rate of drunkenness. And the more removed the individual is from the Jewish community, the more likely he or she will be prone to abuse alcohol and other drugs.

Unfortunately, Jewish immunity is a myth. It is popularly assumed that only "shickuv vi a goyium;" that it is the gentile who is a drunkard. However, alcoholics and drug addicts have always been found in the Jewish community. The alcoholics might not have been seen, but they were present and continue to be present even among some of the most devout Jews; even among Orthodox Rabbis.

Denial continues to be the typical response to addiction within the Jewish community. The myth of Jewish immunity has been an important tool in helping Jewish alcoholics and their families deny that the problem exists. As a result, treatment is not sought. Because Rabbis "know" that Jews are immune, they all too often do not recognize the problem within their congregations nor have they been willing to have synagogues used for alcohol/drug education programs and such twelve step meetings as Alcoholics Anonymous, Narcotics Anonymous, and Al-Anon. Some professionals have likewise had difficulty diagnosing addiction in Jewish clients because they, too, "know" that Jews are immune.

Fortunately, actions are being taken to educate the Jewish community about the dangers of alcoholism and other drug addiction. New scholarship has been able to demonstrate that addiction is a reality. And even those individuals who might wish to cling to the notion that some type of immunity has historically protected Jews cannot easily deny studies which show that alcoholism is on the rise in Israel and is a problem in the United States.

The Federation of Jewish Philanthropies in New York has been a leading voice in educational efforts done to destroy the myth of Jewish immunity. Since 1973, they have published three anthologies devoted to the issue of addiction among Jews: *Judaism and Drugs* (Landman, 1973), *Alcoholism and the Jewish Community* (Blaine, 1980), and *Addictions in the Jewish Community* (Levy & Blume, 1986). Articles in the Jewish Press typically focus on the disease concept of alcoholism and use first person stories of Jews who have recovered from alcoholism and other drug addictions. Frequently, they cite alcoholism even among rabbis to show that one may be a devout Jew and still have a drug problem. These testimonials and other general articles typically stress that denial within the community lengthens the time it takes people to get help.

Jewish Alcoholics, Chemically Dependent Persons, and Significant Others (JACS), a national organization for supporting Jews in recovery programs as well as their families serves not only as a support group, but also holds retreats, publishes a newsletter, and educates rabbis about the problems faced by Jews in recovery. As part of their work, they help Jewish alcoholics become comfortable with the spiritual program of recovery developed by

Alcoholics Anonymous. In order to make Jews more comfortable at AA meetings, they encourage synagogues to provide meeting space for Alcoholics Anonymous, Narcotics Anonymous, Al-Anon, and other recovery programs. More information can be obtained from JACS, 197 E. Broadway, New York, NY 10002.

REFERENCES

Berg, S.L. (1989a) *AA, Spiritual Issues, and the Treatment of Lesbian and Gay Alcoholics.* East Lansing, MI: Michigan State University.

Berg, S.L. (1989b) *Alcoholism and Pastoral Ministry: Readings on Recovery.* Lake Orion, MI: Guest House.

Berg, S.L., D. Finnegan, & E. McNally. (1987) *The NALGAP Annotated Bibliography: Alcoholism, Substance Abuse, and Lesbians/Gay Men.* Ft. Wayne: NALGAP.

Bishop, C. & B. Pittman (1989) *The Annotated Bibliography of Alcoholics Anonymous, 1939-1989.* Wheeling, WV: Bishop of Books.

Blaine, A. (ed.). (1980) *Alcoholism in the Jewish Community.* New York: Federation of Jewish Philanthropies.

Landman, Leo (ed.) (1973) *Judaism and Drugs.* New York: Federation of Jewish Philanthropies.

Levy, S.J. & S. Blume (eds.) (1986) *Addictions in the Jewish Community.* New York: Federation of Jewish Philanthropies.

McNally, E.B. (1989) *Lesbian Recovering Alcoholics in Alcoholics Anonymous: A Qualitative Study of Identity Transformation.* New York: New York University.

Pittman, D.J. & C.R. Snyder (eds.) (1962) *Society, Culture, and Drinking Patterns.* New York: John Wiley and Sons.

Snyder, C.R. (1962) "Culture and Jewish Sobriety: The Ingroup-Outgroup Factor." (pp. 188-225) In Pittman, D.J. & C.R. Snyder (eds.). New York: John Wiley and Sons.

JEWISH ALCOHOLISM
AND
DRUG ADDICTION

1

General Studies

001. (n.a.). (n.d.). *Alcohol and Drug Action Program of Jewish Family Services.* Los Angeles, California: Jewish Community Foundation.

      The program available at Los Angeles' Jewish Family Services.

002. (n.a.). (8 April 1977). "Alcoholism Among Jews? There But Not Acknowledged." *Jewish Record.*

003. (n.a.). (1980). "All About Alcoholism." A. Blaine (ed.), *Alcoholism and the Jewish Community.* (pp. 17-45). New York: Federation of Jewish Philanthropies of New York.

      Gives a brief history of alcohol use and a discussion of current attitudes toward alcohol. Discusses alcohol and youth, ways to overcome alcoholism, and the clergy's role in helping the alcoholic. Jewish alcoholics are not mentioned specifically.

004. Apthorp, S. P. (1985). *Alcohol and Substance Abuse.* Wilton, CT: Morehouse-Barlow.

Describes the minister's dilemma in working with alcoholics and other drug addicts and then explains how the clergy can be a catalyst for change. Techniques clergy can use for creating a treatment network. Jews only mentioned briefly.

005.   Bell, R. G. (1970). *Escape from Addiction*. New York: McGraw-Hill.

Briefly mentions religious and cultural factors which lead to a low rate of alcoholism among Jews.

006.   Bissell, L. & Haberman, P. W. (1984). *Alcoholism in the Professions*. New York: Oxford University Press.

Briefly describes various denominations' responses to alcoholic clergy.

007.   Blume, S. B. (1980). "Alcohol and Its Effects on the Body." A. Blaine (ed.), *Alcoholism and the Jewish Community*. (pp. 47-57). New York: Federation of Jewish Philanthropies of New York.

Overview of medical aspects of alcohol. Jewish alcoholics are not specifically mentioned.

008.   Blume, S. B. & Dropkin, D. (1980). "The Jewish Alcoholic--An Unrecognized Minority." A. Blaine (ed.), *Alcoholism and the Jewish Community*. (pp. 123-133). New York: Federation of Jewish Philanthropies of New York.

That Jewish alcoholics don't exist is a myth.

009.   Blume, S., Dropkin, D., & Sokolow, L. (1984). "A Study of Jewish Alcoholics." *Digest of Alcoholism Therapy and Application*, *3*(4), 19-25.

Originally appeared in *Alcohol, Health, and Research World* (1980) as "The Jewish Alcoholic: A Descriptive Study" 4(4), 21-26.

010. (April, 1986) "Breaking the Silence." *Moment, 11,* 3-5.

011. Cahalan, D., Cisin, I. H., & Crossley, H. M. (1969). *American Drinking Practices: A National Survey of Drinking Behavior and Attitudes.* New Brunswick: Rutgers Center of Alcohol Studies.

Jews drink very little.

012. Clinebell, H. J. (1970). "An Opportunity for the Churches." D. L. Gatlin (ed.), *Attitudes on Alcohol and Drugs.* (pp. 10-13). North Conway, NH: Reporter Press.

Explains the opportunities which churches, temple, and synagogues have for ministering to alcoholics.

013. Clinebell, H. J. (1963). "Philosophical-Religious Factors in the Etiology and Treatment of Alcoholism." *Quarterly Journal of Studies on Alcohol, 24,* 473-488.

Thesis is that "one of the significant factors in the etiology of alcoholism is the vain attempt of the person to satisfy deep religious needs by means of alcohol."

014. (n.a.). (n.d.). "Conquering Alcohol Abuse." In *Conquering Alcohol Abuse.* (pp. 3-4, 7-11). Pasadena, California: Worldwide Church of God.

Information on the low rate of alcoholism among conservative and Orthodox Jews.

015. Courtwright, D. T. & Miller, S. (1986). "Progressivism and Drink: The Social and Photographic Investigations of

James McCook." T. D. Watts (ed.), *Social Thought on Alcoholism.* (pp. 89-108). Malabar, FL: Robert E. Krieger Publishing Company.

Photograph shows the inside of a bar owned by Bernard Kommel, a Russian Jew.

016.   (n.a.). (June 1986). Diagnosis. *Alcoholic Moment Magazine,* 45-47.

Includes information on alcoholic Jews.

017.   Dresner, S.H. (Fall, 1983) "Alcohol and the Jew." *Jewish Information, 4,* 68-71.

018.   Duckat, W. (1981). "Jews and Alcohol." *The Jewish Spectator, 46,* 19-22.

019.   Durkheim, E. (1897). *Le Suicide.* Paris: Alcan.

020.   Engelman, U. Z. (1959). "Review of *Alcohol and the Jews.*" *Jewish Social Studies, 21*(4), 271-272.

Positive review of Charles Snyder's *Alcohol and the Jews.* Sets the work in its historic context.

021.   Ewing, J. A. & Rouse, B. A. (1978). "Drinks, Drinkers, and Drinking." J. A. Ewing & B. A. Rouse (eds.), *Drinking Alcohol in American Society--Issues and Current Research.* (pp. 5-30). Chicago: Nelson-Hall.

Describes the low rate of alcoholism among Jews.

022.   (n.a.). (n.d.). *Exodus Addiction Treatment Programs.* Miami, FL: Exodus.

Describes first treatment center for alcoholic Jews.

023. Falik, A. (1977). "The Problem of Alcoholism." *Public Health*, *19*, 465-466.

024. Fishberg, M. (1905). "Health and Sanitation: New York." C. S. Bernheimer (ed.), *The Russian Jew in the United States*. (pp. 282-303). Philadelphia: John C. Winston.

Sees alcoholism as a growing problem among New York Jews.

025. Ford, J. C. (November 1986). "The Sickness of Alcoholism: Still More Clergy Education?" *Homiletic and Pastoral Review*, 10- 18.

Clergy must cooperate with other professionals in order to help the alcoholic. Briefly mentions that the alcoholics's conduct goes against Christian, Mormon, and Jewish rules of morality.

026. Frankel, L. K. (1905). "Philanthropy: New York." C. S. Bernheimer (ed.), *The Russian Jew in the United States*. (pp. 62- 74). Philadelphia: John C. Winston Company.

Explains that the "instances in which drunkenness lies at the bottom of Jewish dependency are so infrequent that they may be ignored."

027. Fromenson, A. H. (1905). "Amusements and Social Life." C. S. Bernheimer (ed.), *The Russian Jew in the United States*. (pp. 222- 232). Philadelphia: John C. Winston.

As the Jewish population increases, the number of saloons in the neighborhood decreases because Jewish drinking is done at home and on special occasions.

028.   Gallob, B. (8 January 1982). "Yeshiva Drug Addict Challenges View Observant Jews Immune." *Intermountain Jewish News*, 7.

Summarizes A.B. Cohen's "Wanted Help for Orthodox Addicts" which appeared in the *Jewish Observer* in November, 1981. Thesis is that Jews are not immune to alcoholism.

029.   Garber, M. L. (September 23, 1982). "Alcoholism Among the Disabled." *Palos Verdes Peninsula News*, 13.

Describes Marcia Cohen Spiegel's work with Jewish alcoholics.

030.   Gerard, D. L. (116). "Intoxication and Addiction." *Quarterly Journal of Studies on Alcohol*, 4(1955), 689-697. Has never seen any Jewish alcoholics but has seen "not many, but a very evident group of Jews who are opiate addicts."

031.   Gerard, D. L. (1959). "Personality and Social Factors in Intoxication and Addiction." R. G. McCarthy (ed.), *Drinking and Intoxication*. (pp. 298-305). New Haven, CT: College and University Press.

"I have never seen a Jewish alcoholic in a clinic or hospital. I am sure they exist, yet I am confident they are rare. On the other hand, I have seen not many but a very evident group of Jews who are opiate addicts." Article is taken from his "Intoxication and Addiction."

032.   Glassner, B. (1977). "Let's Investigate Jewish Alcoholism." *Sh'ma*, 8(142), 194-195.

Discusses reasons Jewish alcoholism rates are lower than the rate for the overall United States adult population. Describes how Jewish alcoholism is hidden or ignored.

033. Glazer, N. (1952). "Why Jews Stay Sober: Social Scientists Examine Jewish Abstemiousness." *Commentary, 13*(2), 181-186.

Gives explanation of why alcoholism is not a problem in the Jewish Community.

034. Goodwin, D. W. (1984). "Biological Predictors of Problem Drinking." P. M. Miller & T. D. Nirenberg (eds.), *Prevention of Alcohol Abuse.* (pp. 97-118). New York: Plenum Press.

Brief mention is made of Jewish alcoholics.

035. Graunke, D. P. (1976). *The Dilemma of Drugs.* Pasadena: Ambassador College Press.

Cites statistics which show that Jews comprise only 1% of the alcoholics in New York City and concludes that "the Jews have developed their 'winning game' for avoiding alcoholism because their culture has been influenced by the Bible."

036. Hancock, D. C. (1982). "Alcohol and the Church." In E. L. Gomberg, H. R. White, & J. A. Carpenter (eds.), *Alcohol, Science, and Society Revisited.* (pp. 355-370). Ann Arbor, Michigan: The University of Michigan Press.

Only brief mention is made of Jewish alcoholics.

037. Hansen, P. L. (1974). *Alcoholism: The Afflicted and the Affected.* Lake Mills, IA: Graphic.
Focuses on the co-dependency.

038.   Harrison, J. (1977). "Church and Alcoholism: A Growing Involvement." *Alcohol Health and Research World, 1*(4), 2-10.

Explains what various denominations are doing to assist alcoholics. Focuses on Christian denominations, but the percentage of Jewish alcoholics is given.

039.   Hess, D. Y. (1970). "The Frequency of Alcoholism in General Practice." *Family Physician, 1*(1), 3-6.

040.   Hoenig, S. B. (1973). "The Use of Drugs: An Historic Excursion." L. Landman (ed.), *Judaism and Drugs*. (pp. 39-50). New York: Federation of Jewish Philanthropies of New York.

Brief history of drug use giving special attention to Jewish involvement in the drug trade.

041.   Hofstein, S. (1973). "Dealing with Drug Problems in the Jewish Community." L. Landman (ed.), *Judaism and Drugs*. (pp. 223-244). New York: Federation of Jewish Philanthropies of New York.

Argues that the "challenge of the Jewish Community is to find the means of utilizing our own values, traditions, and purposes" to address the growing drug problem.

042.   Hornblass, J. (1980). "Alcohol Abuse--A Jewish Concern." A. Blaine (ed.), *Alcoholism and the Jewish Community*. (pp. 239-247). New York: Federation of Jewish Philanthropies of New York.

Argues that Jews need to recognize addiction as a growing problem.

043. Jewish Telegraphic Agency. (1976). "Expert Says Alcohol Use Growing Among Jews of All Ages." *Community News Reporter*, *15*(12), np.

044. (n.a.). (Fall, 1980). "Jewish Alcoholics." *National Jewish Monthly*, *95*, 54.

045. (n.a.). (24 October 1982). "Jewish Alcoholism is Increasing in Conflict with Tradition. *Democrat and Chronicle*, 1.

046. (n.a.). (n.d.). *Jewish Spirituality in Recovery*. np: np.

Program for one day seminar for Jews in Twelve Step Programs.

047. (n.a.). (26 June 1978). "Jews and Alcoholism: No Cultural Immunity Found" *Medical World News*, 20-21.

Counters the assumption that Jews are culturally immune to alcoholism.

048. (n.a.). (20 September 1978). "Jews Shown not to be 'Immune' to Alcoholism." *National Institute on Alcohol Abuse and Alcoholism Information and Feature Service*, 3.

Argues that Jewish alcoholics are much the same as other alcoholics.

049. Jones, H. (1959). *Alcoholic Addiction: A Psycho-Social Approach to Abnormal Drinking*. London: Tavistock.

Includes section on alcohol use in Orthodox tradition.

050. Kazin, A. (1976) "'The Giant Killer;' Drink and the American Writer." *Commentary*, *61*(3), 44-50.

Describes lives of alcoholic writers.

051.   Keller, M. (1971). "Drunkenness." *Encyclopedia Judaica, 6,* 239+.

052.   Kopf, E. W. (1932). Review of Recent Literature on Alcohol as a Community Health Problem. H. Emerson (ed.), *Alcohol and Man.* (pp. 396-429). New York: MacMillan.

        Cites research which claims that Jews have a lower rate of alcoholism than non-Jews.

053.   (n.a.). (1987). *L'Chaim Retreats.* (np).

        Includes the schedule and handouts for the second annual L'Chaim Retreat.

054.   Landman, L. (1978). "Introduction." L. Landman (ed.), *Judaism and Drugs.* (pp. 17-31). New York: Federation of Jewish Philanthropies of New York.

        Gives a brief history of drug use in Jewish culture.

055.   Levitt, L. (21 June 1977). "Growing Problems Seen in Jewish Alcoholism." *Newsday.*

        Focuses on the issue of assimilation as a cause of Jewish alcoholism.

056.   Levy, S. J. & Rosenwasser, B. G. (1981). *Alcoholism: Is It a Problem in the Jewish Community.* New York: Beth Israel Medical Center.

        Addresses whether alcoholism is a problem in the Jewish community. Gives resources for alcoholics and their families in the New York area.

057.   Lewin, L. (1964). *Phantastica.* London: Routeland, Kegan, Paul.

Explains that the opiate effects of poppies were well known in antiquity. Cites the fact that poppies appear on the bronze coins of the Jewish high priest in 135-106 BCE.

058. Lipman, J. G. (1905). "Rural Settlements: Eastern States." C. S. Bernheimer (ed.), *The Russian Jew in the United States*. (pp. 376-391). Philadelphia: John C. Winston Company.

"Theft and drunkenness are practically unknown in the colonies, although wine and beer are consumed in considerable quantities."

059. Lord, L. (1987). "Coming to Grips with Alcoholism." *U.S. News and World Report*, *103*(22), 56-62.

Brief mention is made of Jews.

060. *Los Angeles Times*. 25 March 1989.

Includes an article which describes a brief which the American Jewish Congress filed on behalf of an atheist who was sentenced to AA. [cited in the *SOS Newsletter* 2.1. (1989): 1]

061. Martin, J. C. (1973). *No Laughing Matter*: *Chalk Talks on Alcohol*. 1946; Cambridge: Harper and Row.

Brief section on how religious background influences drinking.

062. Martin, J. C. (1971). "What is Alcoholism." *NCCA Blue Book*, *23*, 3-16.

Brief mention is made of the fact that Jews don't condone drunkenness.

063. McCarthy, P. D. (1963). "Alcoholism." In E. F. O'Doherty & S. D. McGrath (eds.), *The Priest and Mental Health.* (pp. 136-141). Staten Island, New York: Society of St. Paul.

Briefly mentions that Jews have a low rate of alcoholism.

064. Milt, H. (1976). *Alcoholism: It's Causes and Cure, a New Handbook.* 1969; New York: Charles Scribner's Sons.

Brief section on alcoholism among Jews.

065. Mitelman, B. (October 1977). "Jews Don't Drink--Or Do They?" *Reform Judaism,* 5.

Focuses on denial that Jews drink excessively.

066. Monroe, M. E. & Stewart Jean (1959). *Alcohol Education for the Layman: A Bibliography.* New Brunswick, NJ: Rutgers University Press.

Summarizes Charles R. Snyder's *Alcohol and the Jews.*

067. Mulligan, E. (1971). "Churches and Attitudes Toward Alcohol Use: Introduction." *NCCA Blue Book, 23,* 93-95.

Stresses need for ecumenicalism.

068. Murphy, G. (24 October 1982). "Jewish Alcoholism is Increasing, in Conflict with Tradition." *Democrat and Chronicle,* B5.

Reports that Jewish alcoholism is increasing.

069. (n.a.). (n.d.). *Operation Survival: The Drug and Alcohol Abuse Prevention Program of Crown Heights.* Brooklyn, NY: Operation Survival.

Describes prevention program designed in cooperation between Jewish and black communities in Crown Heights.

070. Patrick, C. H. (1952). *Alcohol, Culture, and Society.* Durham, NC: Duke University Press.

Summarizes previous findings on the rate of alcoholism among Jews.

071. (n.a.). (Fall, 1974). "Physiological Effects: Soldiers Who Take a Nip." *Jewish Observer, 23,* 17.

072. Raymond, I. W. (1927). *The Teaching of the Early Church on the Use of Wine and Strong Drink.* New York: Columbia University Press.

Explains early church teaching on the use of alcohol. Brief mention of Jews.

073. Rea, F. B. (1960). "The Spiritual Approach." *Tomorrow Will Be Sober.* (pp. 183-199). New York: Harper and Row.

Mentions how "rulers of a local synagogue" tried to break up party hosted by St. Matthew.

074. Rosenthal, G. S. (1978). "Preface." L. Landman (ed.), *Judaism and Drugs.* (pp. 13-16). New York: Federation of Jewish Philanthropies of New York.

Argues that drug abuse is also a Jewish problem.

075. Ross, S. G. (June, 1989). *Alcoholism and Problem Drinking Behaviors in Roman Catholic Seminaries.* Illinois School of Professional Psychology,Chicago, Illinois.

Jewish community is discussed in introductory material.

076. Rowe, C. J. (1969). "Alcoholism." In D. L. Farnsworth & F. J. Braceland (eds.), *Psychiatry, the Clergy, and Pastoral Counseling.* (pp. 231-242). Collegeville, Minnesota: St. John's University Press.

     Jewish Family Service Agencies are mentioned as a source for help.

077. Royce, J. E. (1986). "Sin or Solace? Religious Views on Alcohol and Alcoholism." T. D. Watts (ed.), *Social Thought on Alcoholism.* (pp. 53-66). Malabar: Robert E. Krieger Publishing Company.

     Attitudes in various denominations are addressed.

078. Rubington, E. (1972). "The Hidden Alcoholic." *Quarterly Journal of Studies on Alcohol, 33*(3), 667-683.

     Mentions that Orthodox Jews prescribe drinking on religious grounds and in moderation while proscribing intoxication and alcoholism.

079. Ruby, W. (December 1986). "Jews and Drugs." *Hadassah Magazine*, 18-23.

     Focuses on increased use of cocaine and crack in the Jewish Community.

080. Samuelson (1980). *A History of Drink.* London: Trubner. Attributes low rate of alcoholism among Jews to the fact that they are a small, isolated community and need to watch their morals and that they do not "follow avocations which necessitate great physical exertion."

081. (1982). "Selling an Agency-Based Program." *Practice Digest, 5*(2), 6-7.

082. Sherry, G. E. (1956). "Sister Ignatia and the A.A." *Sign,* *35*(10), 9-11.

Mentions that Rosary Hall was built with the help of many AA-alcoholics and with contributions from Protestants, Catholics, and Jews.

083. Snyder, C. R. (1979). "The Rarity of Alcoholism Among Jews: Is It Biological or Socioculturally Determined?" R. M. Goodman & A. G. Motulsky (eds.), *Genetic Diseases Among Ashkenazi Jews.* (pp. 353-362). New York: Rauen.

Gives an overview of studies that demonstrated the rarity of alcoholism among Jews.

084. Sorgen, C. (13 February 1981). "Life on the Rocks: The Jewish Alcoholic." *Baltimore Jewish Times, 40,* 41-45.

Reports on the growing number of Jewish alcoholics and offers suggestions as to how the Jewish community can respond to alcoholism. Brief mention is made of two alcoholics who are orthodox Jewish rabbis.

085. Spencer, J. M. (1979). "West Coast Seminar Lifts Veil of Denial." *NCA News: From the Alcoholism Council of South Bay, 2*(1), 1.

Attention is given to the argument that the "dis-ease" of spiritual emptiness found in the Jewish community contributed to alcoholism.

086. Spencer, J. M. (Spring 1979). "West Coast Seminar Lifts Veil of Denial." *Alcoholism and the Jewish Community Newsletter,* 1-3.

087. Spiegel, M. C. (Autumn 1987). "Beyond Inclusion: Redefining the Jewish Family." *Genesis 2,* 14-16.

Argues that the generally accepted model of the Jewish family is unworkable because it doesn't acknowledge the existence of alcoholism, domestic violence, incest, gay men, lesbians, and single people.

088.   Spiegel, M. C. (December 1978). "Jewish Alcoholism Growing Problem for Community." *Los Angeles Jewish Community Bulletin*, 3.

089.   Spiegel, M.C. (1981) "Jews and Alcoholism." *Jewish Digest*, *26*(6), 6-12.

Reprint of "The Wrath of Grapes: Jews and Booze" which appeared in *Hadassah Magazine*, 16-17, 37.

090.   Spiegel, M. C. (September 19, 1980). "New Light Shed on Jewish Alcoholics." *Los Angeles B'nai B'rith Messenger*, 19.

Summarizes *The Heritage of Noah* and Sheila Blume and others' "The Jewish Alcoholic."

091.   Spiegel, M. C. (November 1980). "The Wrath of Grapes: Jews and Booze." *Hadassah Magazine*, 16-17, 37.

Reviews history of alcohol and discusses possible causes of Jewish alcoholism.

092.   Spitzer, B. (1987). "Jewish Board of Education Develops Substance Abuse Curriculum." *JACS Journal*, *4*(1), 1. Reports on a drug education program designed by the New York Jewish Board of Education.

093.   Stein, R. H. (1975). "Wine-Drinking in New Testament Time." *Christianity Today*, *19*(19), 9-11.

Paragraph describes the Jewish definition of wine.

094. Steinhardt, D. (1988). "Alcoholism: The Myth of Jewish Immunity." *Psychology Today*, 22, 10.

Presents view that alcoholic Jews are not rare.

095. Steinman, D. (1989). "Jewish Concepts and Recovery from Chemical Dependency." *JACS Journal*, 6(1), 2-4.

Describes how the addict's personality affects his/her spirituality.

096. Steinman, D. (1984). "Meditations." *JACS*, 1(2), 6.

Meditation which focuses on the fact that "Judaism is not a religion of blind acceptance of dogma" and that "there is potentially no difference between our 'secular' and our 'religious' lives." Growth in service to God is stressed.

097. Stewart, D. A. (1960). "Religion, Science, and AA." In D. A. Stewart, *Thirst for Freedom*. (pp. 133-142). Center City, MN: Hazelden.

Analyzes the religious elements within AA and demonstrates how non-Christians can understand the steps within the context of their own traditions.

098. Straus, R. (1951). "Non-Addictive Pathological Drinking Patterns of Homeless Men." *Quarterly Journal of Studies on Alcohol*, 12(4), 601-611.

Argues that skid row "alcoholics" should more often be classified as pathological rather than alcoholic drinkers. Jews mentioned.

099. Thorner, I. (1953). "Ascetic Protestantism and Alcoholism." *Psychiatry*, 16(2), 167-176.

Examines the evidence which suggests that there is a relationship between alcoholism and religious denominations.

100.   Trainin, I. N. (1973). "The Role of the Commission on Synagogue Relations in Drug Programs." L. Landman (ed.), *Judaism and Drugs*. (pp. 51-58). New York: Federation of Jewish Philanthropies of New York.

History of the role of the Commission on Synagogue Relations in Drug Programs.

101.   Trainin, I. N. (1982). "Alcoholism in the Jewish Community." I. N. Trainin (ed.), *A Generation of Service*. New York: Federation of Jewish Philanthropies.

Overview of issues that face Jewish alcoholics

102.   Trainin, I. N. (1986). "Alcoholism in the Jewish Community." S. J. Levy & S. B. Blume (eds.), *Addictions in the Jewish Community*. (pp. 15-27). New York: Federation of Jewish Philanthropies of New York.

Reprinted from Issac N. Trainin (1982) *A Generation of Service* New York: Federation of Jewish Philanthropies.

103.   W.S.G. (1974). "Alcoholism." In I. Singer (ed.), *The Jewish Encyclopedia* (pp. 333-334) New York: Funk and Wagnalls.

Argues that alcoholism is rare among Jews.

104.   Warren, M. R. (1980). "Alcohol and the Jewish Community." A. Blaine (ed.), *Alcoholism and the Jewish Community*. (pp. 223-229). New York: Federation of Jewish Philanthropies of New York.

Provides general criteria for school based alcohol education programs.

105. Watts, T. D. & Wright, R. J., eds. (1983). *Black Alcoholism: Toward a Comprehensive Understanding.* Springfield: Charles C. Thomas.

Appendix lists resources for Jewish alcoholics.

106. Weiss, C. (6 March 1981). "Help Is Available for Alcoholics." *Phoenix Jewish News*, *6*, 6-7.

Where Jewish alcoholics and their families can get help in the Phoenix area.

107. Weiss, L. (1977). "We Accept Drinking But Not Drunkenness." *Sh'ma*, *8*(142), 192-194.

Explains higher than expected rate of alcoholism among Jews.

108. Yablonsky, L. (1967). *Synanon: The Tunnel Back.* Baltimore: Penguin.

Brief section devoted to "Patterns of Religion" mentions Jews.

109. Youcha, G. (December, 1979) "The Jewish Alcoholic: From Kiddish to Cocktails." *National Jewish Monthly*, *94*, 16-18.

2

Empirical Studies

110.   Adlaf, E. M., Smart, R. G., & Tan, S. H. (1989). "Ethnicity and Drug Use: A Critical Look." *International Journal of the Addictions, 24*(1), 1-18.

Found that "the significant zero-order ethnicity effect for alcohol use did not attenuate after controlling for background variables" and that "this relationship was not conditional upon other independent variables." For other drugs, "the significant zero-order ethnicity effect was found to be spurious or conditional."

111.   Bacon, S. D. (1951). "Studies of Drinking in Jewish Culture: General Introduction." *Quarterly Journal of Studies on Alcohol, 12*(3), 444-450.

A general introduction to Charles R. Snyder's Studies of Drinking in Jewish Culture." Scientific methodology is explained and then related to the study of alcoholism.

112.   Bailey, M. B., Haberman, P. W., & Alkene, H. (1965). "The Epidemiology of Alcoholism in an Urban Residential Area." *Quarterly Journal of Studies on Alcohol, 26*(1), 19-40.

Two percent of the sample were Jewish.

113. Bales, R. F. (1962). "Attitudes Toward Drinking in the Irish Culture." In D. J. Pittman & C. R. Snyder (eds.), *Society, Culture, and Drinking Patterns*. (pp. 157-187). New York: John Wiley and Sons.

A revised and shortened version of chapter 4 of Bales' *The "Fixation Factor" in Alcohol Addiction*.

114. Bernheimer, C. S., ed. (1905). *The Russian Jew in the United States: Studies of Social Conditions in New York, Philadelphia, and Chicago, with a Description of Rural Settlements, Philadelphia*. np: J.C. Winston Co.

Dominant theme in this collection of essays is the lack of drunkenness among immigrant Russian Jews.

115. Bernheimer, C. S. (1905). "Health and Sanitation: Philadelphia." C. S. Bernheimer (ed.), *The Russian Jew in the United States*. (pp. 304-317). Philadelphia: John C. Winston.

Found that diseases to alcoholic excess "are rarely met with among the Jewish poor."

116. Blume, S. B. & Dropkin, D. (1980). "The Jewish Alcoholic: An Unrecognized Minority." *Journal of Psychiatric Treatment and Evaluation*, 2, 1-4.

Survey of 100 Jewish alcoholics. Focus on special problems and defence mechanisms.

117. Brock, E. W., Cochran, J. K., & Beeghley, L. (1987). "Moral Messages: The Relative Influence of Denomination on the Religiosity-Alcohol Relationship." *The Sociological Quarterly*, 28(1), 89-103.

Religiosity and alcohol use is greater in proscriptive than nonproscriptive religions and the religiosity-misuse relationship is weaker than the religiosity-use relationship.

118.   Feebey, F. E., Mindlin, D. F., Minear, V. H., & Short, E. E. (1955). "The Challenge of the Skid Row Alcoholic." *Quarterly Journal of Studies on Alcohol, 16*(4), 643-667.

Study of differences between chronic alcoholics sentenced to a workhouse and those who voluntarily admitted themselves to a clinic. In this study, 60% of the individuals were Protestants, 24% were Catholics, 2% were Jews, and 14% were unaffiliated.

119.   Feldman, J., Su, W. H., Kaley, M. M., & Kissin, B. (1975). "Skid Row and Inner-City Alcoholics: A Comparison of Drinking Patterns and Medical Problems." *Quarterly Journal of Studies on Alcohol, 35*(2), 565-576.

2.1% of the skid row alcoholics and 3.0% of the inner-city alcoholics were Jewish.

120.   Galdi, J. & Bonato, R. R. (1981). "Common Genetic Mechanisms in Alcoholism and Psychiatric Disorders: Negative Evidence from a Study of Ethnic Group Patients." *Alcoholism: Clinical and Experiment Research, 5*(3), 366-371.

Testing ethnic populations with low rates of alcoholism, the authors "predicted that decreased alcoholism would be substituted for by increased psychiatric disorder." Results did not support this hypothesis.

121.   Glassner, B. (1984). "Alcohol Abuse as a State: Illustrations of the 'Structuration Model'." *Journal of Drug Issues, 14*(1), 95- 107.

"Centers on the derivations of social meanings of objects and behaviors that are neglected through the use of other strategies" and focuses on "drinking related expressions among Orthodox and non-Orthodox Jews, focusing on avoidance of alcohol problems."

122.   Glassner, B. & Berg, B. (1984). "Social Locations and Interpretations: How Jews Define Alcoholism." *Journal of Studies on Alcohol, 45*(1), 16-25.

Study of 88 Jews living in central New York state. Found that "Orthodox Jews tend to offer disease definitions of alcoholism...whereas Reform and nonpracticing Jews define alcoholism in terms of psychological dependency and view suspected alcoholics with condemnation and blame."

123.   Goldstein, S. (1964). *The Greater Providence Jewish Community: A Population Survey*. Providence: by the author.

124.   Hyde, R. W. & Chisholm, R. M. (1944). "Studies in Medical Sociology. III. The Relationship of Mental Disorders to Race and Nationality." *New England Journal of Medicine, 231*, 612-618.

Studied selected people for induction to the armed forces to determine the rate of mental illness in the general population. Chronic alcoholism among Jews is mentioned.

125.   Jacobson, G. R. & Lindsay, D. (1980). "Screening for Alcohol Problems Among the Unemployed." M. Galanter (ed.), *Currents in Alcoholism. 7* (pp. 357-371). New York: Grune and Stratton.

Reports on a study taken of welfare recipients applying for CETA benefits at the Milwaukee office of Jewish Vocational Service from March 1, 1978 to September 30,

1978. The following characteristics of the unemployed population were studied: sex, age, education, and racial-ethnic identification.

126. Kane, R. L. & Patterson, E. (1972). "Drinking Attitudes and Behavior of High School Students in Kentucky." *Quarterly Journal of Studies on Alcohol, 33*(3), 635-646.

Report on a survey of 119,929 Kentucky high school students of whom half were non-drinkers and 3% were heavy drinkers. "The religious affiliation reported by the respondents were 47% Protestant, 31% Catholic, 2% Jewish, and 17% other (of which a substantial proportion is probably other Protestant religions); 4% reported no religious affiliation."

127. Levy, K. (1905). "Health and Sanitation: Chicago." C. S. Bernheimer (ed.), *The Russian Jew in the United States.* (pp. 318- 333). Philadelphia: John C. Winston Company.

In the west side district of Chicago which contains about 30,000 Russian Jews, "Temperance rules supreme." Except for prohibition districts, there are fewer saloons than in other neighborhoods.

128. Liberson, D. M. (1956). Causes of Death Among Jews in New York City in 1953. *Jewish Social Studies, 18*(2), 83-117.

Found that "statistics on all diseases caused partly or wholly by alcoholism confirm its low incidence among Jews."

129. Malzberg, B. (1963). *Mental Health of Jews in New York State: A Study of First Admissions to Hospitals for Mental Disease, 1949-1950.* Albany: Research Foundation for Mental Hygiene.

Malzberg analyzes the 27 cases of Jewish first admissions for alcoholic psychoses.

130. Mayer, J., Needham, M. A., & Myerson, D. J. (1965). "Contact and Initial Attendance at an Alcoholism Clinic." *Quarterly Journal of Studies on Alcohol, 26*(3), 480-485.

Studied characteristics of individuals who contact an alcoholism clinic to determine differences between those who appear for their initial appointment and those who do not. Contact group included 74% Catholic, 25% Protestants, and 1% Jewish. Religious factors were not analyzed.

131. Meyers, A. R., Hingson, R., Mucatel, M., Heeren, T., & Goldman, E. (1985). "Social Epidemiology of Alcohol Use by Urban Older Adults." *International Journal of Aging and Human Development, 21*(1), 49-59.

Found that "women, blacks, Jews, widows and widowers, the foreign-born, those with low levels of formal education, and those 75 years or older" drink the least.

132. Milman, D.H. & W.H. Su. *Patterns of Drug Use Among University Students*

Correlates marijuana intake with Jewish background.

133. Moros, N. (1942). "The Alcoholic Personality: A Statistical Study." *Quarterly Journal of Studies on Alcohol, 3*(1), 45-49.

Study of admissions to the U.S. Veterans Administration Facility in Northport, RI between January 1, 1936 to July 1, 1939. Found that chronic alcoholism was rare among Jews.

134.   Myerson, A. (1941). "Neuroses and Alcoholism Among the Jews." *Medical Leaves, 3*, 104-107.

135.   Myerson, A. (1944). "The Treatment of Alcohol Addiction in Relation to the Prevention of Inebriety." *Quarterly Journal of Studies on Alcohol, 5*(2), 189-199.

Found few alcoholics among Jews.

136.   Parsons, T. & Alger, B. C. (1979). "Characteristics of Drug-Overdosed Patients and Supplementary Treatment Needs." *The Journal of Pastoral Care, 33*(2), 88-95.

Characteristics of emergency room patients who had overdosed on drugs. Types of drugs used as well as religious affiliation were included. Suggestions are given as to how hospital chaplains can effectively minister to such patients.

137.   Perkins, H. W. (1985). "Religious Traditions, Parents, and Peers as Determinants of Alcohol and Drug Use Among College Students." *Review of Religious Research, 27*(1), 15-31.

Examines the relationship between religiosity and drinking/drug use among college students in the context of family background and peer relationships. Large number of Jewish students in the study.

138.   Rice, C. G. & Shaw, J. S. (1984). "Male and Female Applicants for Alcoholism Treatment: A Study of Differential Staff Attitudes." *Journal of Drug Issues, 114*(4), 677-686.

Studied staff attitudes on who were most desirable candidates for treatment.

139. Rosenbloom, J. R. (1959). "Notes on Jewish Drug Addicts." *Psychological Reports*, *5*, 769-772.

"The characteristics of 32 Jewish drug addicts in residence at the U.S.P.H. Hospital during Spring, 1958, indicated that they were introduced to drugs at a fairly early age, had poor relationships with their fathers, were the youngest or eldest child, came predominantly from New York City, and were unable to maintain a successful marital relationship. The majority smoked marijuana or used heroin. Length of addiction averaged was 11 years."

140. Scaturo, D. J. & LeSure, K. B. (1985). "Symptomatic Correlates of Alcohol Abuse as a Presenting Problem." *Journal of Clinical Psychology*, 41(1), 118-123.

Assessed the relationship of self reported symptoms of psychopathology to alcohol abuse. Of the participants, 48.6% were Catholic, 41.7% were Protestants, 2.8% were Jewish, and 5.6% were of some other denomination.

141. Seidman, H., Stellman, S. D., & Mushinski, M. H. (1982). "Different Perspective on Breast Cancer Risk Factors: Some Implications of the Nonattributable Risk." *CA-A Cancer Journal for Clinicians*, *32*(5), 301-313.

Being Jewish and having daily alcohol consumption were both factors for placing a woman at higher risk for developing breast cancer.

142. Skolnick, J. S. (1954). "A Study of the Relation of Ethnic Background to Arrest for Inebriety." *Quarterly Journal of Studies on Alcohol*, *15*(4), 622-630.

Study of drunk driving arrests made in New Haven, CT during July, 1951.

143.   Snyder, C. (1958). *Alcohol and the Jews: A Cultural Study of Drinking and Sobriety*. Glencoe, IL: Free Press.

Investigates the rate of alcoholism and the drinking practices of Jews. This book is based on his dissertation.

144.   Snyder, C. R. (1958). *Alcohol and the Jews: A Cultural Study of Drinking and Sobriety*. Rutgers Center of Alcohol Studies, New Brunswick.

Reprinted as *Alcohol and the Jews*. Carbondale: Southern Illinois University Press, 1958. It was the first published version of Snyder's dissertation.

145.   Snyder, C. (1954). *Culture and Sobriety: A Study of Drinking Patterns and Sociocultural Factors Related to Sobriety Among Jews*. New Haven, CT: Yale University.

Investigates the rate of alcoholism and the drinking practices of Jews. The dissertation was published as *Alcohol and the Jews*.

146.   Spiegel, M. C. (1979). *The Heritage of Noah: Alcoholism in the Jewish Community*. Hebrew Union College.

Gives an overview of attitudes toward strong drink in classical Jewish literature, historical perspectives on Jewish attitudes toward drinking, and the disease concept of alcoholism. Presents the findings of her study of Jewish alcoholics and proposes a Jewish approach to the treatment of alcoholism.

147.   Straus, R. (1951). "A Note on the Religion of Male Alcoholism Clinic Patients." *Quarterly Journal of Studies on Alcohol, 12*(3), 560-561.

Reports on the percentage of Jewish alcoholics in a recent study supporting the idea that the rate of alcoholism is lower in the Jewish community than in the general population.

148. Vyvial, T. M. & Hecht, F. (1982). "Alcoholic Cirrhosis in Ashkenazi Jews and HLA." *Lancet*, 2(8293), 326.

Suggests that the low level of HLA-B8 among Ashkenazi Jews might contribute to the low rate of alcoholism among this population. For response, see M.M. Glatt's "Alcoholic Cirrhosis in Jews" *Lancet* (1982) 2: 558.

149. Waldorf, D. (1973). "Women vs. Men." *Careers in Dope*. (pp. 159-177). Englewood Cliffs, NJ: Prentice Hall.

Conducted "to determine the specific differences between men and women addicts aside from obvious sex and role differences." Major religious group was Catholic, but 39% of the respondents were Protestants and 3% percent were Jewish.

150. Waldorf, D. (1974). "Women vs. Men." P. Ferguson, T. Lennox, & D. J. Lettieri (eds.), *Drugs and Sex*. (pp. 69-71). Rockville, MD: National Institute on Drug Abuse.

Summary of Waldorf's article of the same title which appeared in *Careers in Dope*, Englewood Cliffs, NJ: Prentice Hall, 1973.

151. Wechsler, H. & McFadden, M. (1979). "Drinking Among College Students in New England: Extent, Social Correlates and Consequences of Alcohol Use." *Journal of Studies on Alcohol*, 40(11), 969-996.

Found a negative correlation between drinking and attendance at religious services.

152. Wechsler, H., Thum, D., Demone Jr., H. W., & Dwinnell, J. (1972). "Social Characteristics and Blood Alcohol Levels." *Quarterly Journal of Studies on Alcohol, 33*(1), 132-147.

Found that "in 6,266 patients admitted to an emergency hospital service, blood alcohol levels were significantly related to sex, age, marital status, and religious-ethnic background, but not social class."

153. Weshler, H. W., Thum, D., Demone, H. W., & Kasey, E. H. (1970). "Religious-Ethnic Difference in Alcohol Consumption." *Journal of Health and Social Behavior, 11*(1), 21-29.

Sampled 8,461 patients admitted to an emergency room to determine alcohol use. Results reported in terms of Catholics, Protestants, Jews, and Negroes.

154. Whitehead, P. C. (1969). *Drug Use Among Adolescent Students in Halifax*. Halifax: Youth Agency, Province of Nova Scotia.

In this study, Whitehead found that in a survey of 7th, 9th, 11th, and 12th graders, 39% of the Catholics, 41% of the Protestants, 52% of the Jews, and 41% of those who had no religious affiliation were drinkers.

155. Wolff, P. (1981). "Studies on Ethnic Differences." *Alcoholism: Clinical and Experimental Research, 5*(3), 444-447.

Mention is made of alcohol flushing in Sephardic Jews.

156. Wolff, S. & Holland, L. (1964). "A Questionnaire Follow-Up of Alcoholic Patients." *Quarterly Journal of Studies on Alcohol, 25*(1), 108-118.

Follow-up study done of patients discharged from a Cape Town hospital for alcoholics from March 1959-August 1961. Of those clients who were members of the Dutch Reformed Church, "26 were abstinent and 11 [were] drinking; Church of England, 17 and 2; Protestants, 16 and 3; Roman Catholic, 9 and 2; Jewish, 1 and 1; other, 4 and 0."

3

Theoretical Studies

157. Bainton, R. H. (1945). "The Churches and Alcohol."
      Quarterly Journal of Studies on Alcohol, 6(1), 45-58.

      Was also published in *Alcohol, Science, and Society* without
      the notes.

158. Bainton, R. H. (1989). "The Churches and Alcohol." S. L.
      Berg (ed.), *Alcoholism and Pastoral Ministry*. (pp. 18-34).
      Lake Orion, MI: Guest House.

      Reprinted from *Quarterly Journal of Studies on Alcohol* 6
      (1945): 45-58.

159. Bainwol, S. & Gressard, C. F. (1985). "Incidence of Jewish
      Alcoholism: A Review of the Literature." *Journal of Drug
      Education, 15*(3), 217-224.

      Comparison of methodology and conclusions of nine studies
      published between 1970 and 1983 on the rate of alcoholism
      in the Jewish community. Authors concluded that the better
      studies showed that the rate of alcoholism among Jews was
      still lower than the general population, but they predicted
      that assimilation would cause an increase in the rate of
      alcoholism.

160. Baird, E. G. (1944). "The Alcohol Problem and the Law." *Quarterly Journal of Studies on Alcohol, 4*(4), 535-556.

     Traces a history of laws and customs concerning the manufacture and use of alcohol. Gives special attention to ancient Hebrew law as well as to ecclesiastical law in the middle ages.

161. Bales, R. F. (1946). "Cultural Differences in Rates of Alcoholism." *Quarterly Journal of Studies on Alcoholism, 6*, 480- 498.

     Argues that there are three ways in which a culture can influence rates of alcoholism: (1) "the degree in which the culture operates to bring about acute needs for adjustment...in its members," (2) "the sort of attitudes [it has] toward drinking," and (3) "the degree to which the culture provides suitable substitute means of satisfaction." Judaism receives special emphasis.

162. Bales, R. F. (1959). "Cultural Differences in Rates of Alcoholism." In R. G. McCarthy (ed.), *Drinking and Intoxication.* (pp. 263-277). New Haven: Yale Center of Alcohol Studies.

     Reprinted from the *Quarterly Journal of Studies on Alcohol* (1946) 6: 480-498.

163. Blaine, A. (ed.) (1980). *Alcoholism in the Jewish Community.* New York: Commission on Synagogue Relations.

     Collection of essays on Jewish alcoholism and other drug addiction.

164.   Brauer, E. (1942). "The Jews of Afghanistan: An Anthropological Report." *Jewish Social Studies*, 4(2), 121-138.

Money-changing and the trade in drugs, which were traditional vocations among the Jews in the Orient.

165.   Cheinisse, L. (1908). "La Race Juive Jouit-elle d'une Immunite a L'egard de L'Alcoolisme?" ["Does the Jewish Race Enjoy an Immunity with Respect to Alcoholism?"]. *Semaine Medicale, 28*, 613- 615.

166.   Cohen, A. (1973). "Why Drugs?" L. Landman (ed.), *Judaism and Drugs*. (pp. 83-94). New York: Federation of Jewish Philanthropies of New York.

Jewish law would prohibit drug use even if drugs were legal.

167.   Cohen, H. H. (1974). *The Drunkenness of Noah*. University of Alabama.

"Discovered that Noah's nakedness was directly related to his drunkenness and his nakedness formed an integral aftermath of the flood story; and that their significance could be appreciated only by probing into the conditions that precipitated the flood."

168.   Davos, R.A. (June, 1990)   "A Jewish Component for Chemical Dependency Prevention Programs in Jewish Settings." manuscript.

Summary of proposed rabbinical thesis concerning myth that Jews have low rate of alcoholism.

169. Delorme, M. F. (1984). "Aspects Etiopothogeniques de l'Alcoolisation et de l'Alcoolisme." *Alcoologie.* (pp. 123-130). Riom, Cedex, France: Riom Laboratoires.

Investigates internal factors involved in the etiology and pathogenesis of alcohol intoxication.

170. Delorme, M. F. (1984). "L'alcool: Quelques Reperes Dans le Temps et l'Espace." *Alcoologie.* (pp. 7-15). Riom, Cedex, France: Riom Laboratoires.

Traces the history of alcohol use in France from 5 BCE to the present. Concludes that even if wine has lost much of its sacred value, its symbolic value and social function remains strong.

171. Diskind, M. H. (1970). "The Jewish Drug Addict--A Challenge to the Jewish Community." G. S. Rosenthal (ed.), *The Jewish Family in a Changing World.* (pp. 122-135). Cranbury, NJ: Thomas Yoseloff.

Jews are not immune to addiction.

172. Diskind, Z. A. (1953). *A Psych-Cultural Investigation of Jewish Drinking Habits and Attitudes.* Portland: np.

173. Douglas, M. (1987). "A Distinctive Anthropological Perspective." in M. Douglas (ed.), *Constructive Drinking.* (pp. 3-15). Cambridge, Massachusetts: Cambridge University Press.

Distance from traditional orthodoxy and not assimilation accounts for the increase of alcoholism in the Jewish community.

174. Drazin, N. (1973). "Halakhic Attitudes and Conclusions to the Drug Problem and its Relationship to Cigarette

Smoking." L. Landman (ed.), *Judaism and Drugs*. (pp. 71-81). New York: Federation of Jewish Philanthropies of New York.

Talmudic dictum forbids the use of narcotic drugs and use of tobacco.

175.   Dulfano, C. (1980). "The Impact of Alcoholism on Jewish Family Life." A. Blaine (ed.), *Alcoholism and the Jewish Community*. (pp. 231-237). New York: Federation of Jewish Philanthropies of New York.

How the alcoholic's behavior affects other family members. Special emphasis to Jewish families.

176.   Fishberg, M. (1911). *The Jews: A Study of Race and Environment*. New York: Walter Scott Publishing Company.

Argues that contemporary Jews abstain from alcohol because ancient Jews drank excessively and because of their religious beliefs concerning hygiene. Social class or geographic location have little affect on Jewish alcoholism.

177.   Flasher, L. V. & Maisto, S. A. (1984). "Review of Theory and Research on Drinking Patterns Among Jews." *Journal of Nervous and Mental Disease, 172*(10), 596-603.

Summarizes theories advanced to explain the drinking patterns among Jews. Reveals substantial methodological and interpretive problems that challenge the conclusions which have been generally accepted.

178.   Glassner, B. & Berg, B. (1980). "How Jews Avoid Alcohol Problems." *American Sociological Review, 45*, 647-664.

Offers four theories as to why Jews avoid alcohol problems: (1) association of alcoholism with non-Jews, (2) integration of moderate drinking norms, (3) restriction of most adult relationships to other moderate drinkers, and (4) techniques to avoid excessive drinking under social pressure.

179. Glassner, B. & Berg, B. (1985). "Jewish Americans and Alcohol: Processes of Avoidance and Definition." In L. A. Bennett & G. M. Ames (eds.), *American Experience with Alcohol.* (pp. 93-107). New York: Plenum Press.

Explains "four protective processes that appear to contribute to the avoidance of alcohol abuse by American Jews." Significant differences in attitudes toward alcoholism and alcoholics with the Jewish community are also addressed.

180. Glatt, M. M. (1970). "Alcoholism and Drug Dependence Amongst Jews." *British Journal of Addiction, 64*(314), 297-304.

Comments on the low rates of alcoholism among Jews as well as on reports of the higher rates of addiction to drugs other than alcohol.

181. Glatt, M. M. (1980). "Alcoholism and Drug Dependence Amongst Jews." A. Blaine (ed.), *Alcoholism and the Jewish Community.* (pp. 187-201). New York: Federation of Jewish Philanthropies of New York.

Reprinted from the *British Journal of Addiction* (1970) 64.314, 297-304.

182. Glatt, M. M. (1982). "Alcoholic Cirrhosis in Jews." *Lancet, 2,* 558.

Response to T.M. Vyvial (1982) "Alcoholic Cirrhosis in Ashkenazi Jews" *Lancet* 2.8293, 325. Argues for a socio-cultural explanation for the low rate of alcoholism among Jews.

183.   Glatt, M. M. (1973). "Les Alcooliques et Autres Toxicomanes Juifs Dans La Region De Londres" ["Jewish Alcoholics and Addicts in the London Area"]. *Toxicomanes*, 6(1), 33-39.

Concludes that alcoholism among middle class Jews is "a not uncommon occurrence." Jewish alcoholics did not have strong ties to family and Jewish cultural tradition.

184.   Glatt, M. M. (1975). "Jewish Alcoholics and Addicts in the London Area." *Mental Health and Society*, 2, 168-174.

Reprinted from *Toxicomanes* (1973) 6.1: 33-39.

185.   Goodwin, D. (1979). "Protective Factors in Alcoholism." *Drug and Alcohol Dependence*, 4, 99-100.

Claims Orientals and Jews have physiological protection against heavy drinking.

186.   Greenwald, R. (1980). "Chassidim and Alcoholism--The Fortunate Contradiction." A. Blaine (ed.), *Alcoholism and the Jewish Community*. (pp. 249-253). New York: Federation of Jewish Philanthropies of New York.

Argues that while alcoholism is increasing in the Jewish Community as a whole the Chassidic Community has not shared in this trend.

187.   Gressard, C. E. & Bainwol, S. "Jewish Drinking Practices: Implications and Prevention."

Reviews the literature that appears to provide Jews with their 'immunity' and discusses how these factors may be applied to prevention programs.

188. Hait, P. L. (1980). "Alcoholism as Reflected in Jewish Tradition." A. Blaine (ed.), *Alcoholism in the Jewish Community.* (pp. 89-99). New York: Federation of Jewish Philanthropies of New York.

Describes the theological basics for the strong Jewish tradition against drunkenness.

189. Herrington, R. (1987). "Alcohol Abuse and Alcohol Dependence: Treatment and Rehabilitation." R. E. Herrington, G. R. Jacobson, & D. G. Benzer (eds.), (pp. 180-218). St. Louis: Warren G. Green, Inc.

Argues "with increasing tendency for intermarriage and cultural assimilation, one is seeing a rising incidence of alcoholism" among Jews.

190. Hewitt, T. F. (1980). *A Biblical Perspective on the Use and Abuse of Alcohol and Other Drugs.* np.

Explains biblical passages on alcohol use. Gives a brief history of alcohol use from biblical times to the present. Section on alcohol use among the Hebrews is included.

191. Hoenig, S. B. (1980). "Alcoholism in the Jewish Community--An Historic Perspective." A. Blaine (ed.), *Alcoholism in the Jewish Community.* (pp. 101-119). New York: Federation of Jewish Philanthropies of New York.

Argues that while Jewish tradition never argued for abstinence, drunkenness was forbidden.

192. Jackson, J. K. & Connor, R. (1953). "Attitudes of the Parents of Alcoholics, Moderate Drinkers and Nondrinkers Towards Drinking." *Quarterly Journal of Studies on Alcohol, 14*(4), 596- 613.

Investigates attitudes of non-drinkers and alcoholics by placing emphasis on the family rather than broader cultural categories. Summary of Jewish drinking practices is given.

193.   Keller, M. (1970). "The Great Jewish Drink Mystery." *British Journal of Addiction, 64*(314), 287-296.

Argues that the Jewish drink mystery is not the low rate of alcoholism, but how Jews moved from a tradition of drunkenness to one of sobriety.

194.   Kerr, N. (1888). *Inebriety, Its Etiology, Pathology Treatment and Jurisprudence.* London: Lewis.

Race and hygiene are attributed to non-existence of alcoholism among Jews.

195.   Kissin, B. (1983). "The Disease Concept of Alcoholism." in R. Smart, F. B. Glasser, Y. Israel, H. Kalant, R. E. Popham, & W. Schmidt (eds.), *Research Advances in Alcohol and Drug Problems: Volume 7.* (pp. 93-126). New York, New York: Plenum Press.

Suggests "a formula called the 'psychological principle' which stated that the degree of psychopathology associated with the development of alcohol dependence or any form of drug addiction, was inversely related to the level of acceptance of a given type of drug abuse in a given individual's subculture." Alcoholic Orthodox Jews would rate high on the scale.

196.   Landman, L. (ed.) (1973). *Judaism and Drugs.* New York, New York: Federation of Jewish Philanthropies of New York.

Includes essays on alcoholism and other drug addiction.

197. Leiberman, L. (1986). Defining Jewish Alcoholism. S. J. Levy & S. B. Blume (eds.), *Addictions in the Jewish Community*. (pp. 29-42). New York: Federation of Jewish Philanthropies of New York.

Examines "the meaning and consequences of deviant drinking practices among Jews and the relationship of this deviant drinking to the definition of alcoholism among Jews."

198. LeVann, L. J. (1953). "A Clinical Survey of Alcoholics." *Canadian Medical Association Journal, 69*(6), 584-588.

Concludes that Jews and Chinese, which have a strong figure in the biological father, tend to have low rates of alcoholism.

199. Levine, H. (1987). "The Alternative Economy of Alcohol in the Chiapas Highlands." in M. Douglas (ed.), *Constructive Drinking*. (pp. 250-269). Cambridge, Massachusetts: Cambridge University Press.

Describes Jewish involvement in *Propinacja*, the monopoly on the manufacture and distribution of alcohol in eighteenth century Poland.

200. Levy, S. J. (1982). "Dealing with Denial: Alcoholism Among Jews." *Bulletin of Social Psychology and Substance Abuse, 1*, 55-58.

Notes myth of Jewish alcoholism and how myth adversely affects Jewish recovery.

201. Levy, S. J. (1986). "Practical Aspects of Outpatient Psychotherapy with Substance Abusers." S. J. Levy & S. B. Blume (eds.), *Addictions in the Jewish Community*. (pp.

297-313). New York: Federation of Jewish Philanthropies of New York.

Presents traps into which a psychotherapist might fall when dealing with individuals addicted to drugs. Spiritual aspects of clients lives are mentioned.

202.   Levy, S. J. & Blume, S. B., eds. (1986). *Addiction in the Jewish Community.* New York: Federation of Jewish Philanthropies of New York.

Includes essays on Jewish alcoholism and other drug addiction.

203.   Liebermann, L. (1987). "Jewish Alcoholism and the Disease Concept." *Journal of Psychology and Judaism, 11,* 165-180.

204.   Lloyd, A. (1984). "Angel Dust: A Religious Dilemma." *American Zionist Quarterly Review, 96*(3), 6-18.

205.   May, G. G. (1988). *Addiction and Grace.* San Francisco: Harper and Row.

Uses Jewish, Christian, and Buddhist scripture to explain the nature of the grace needed to overcome addiction.

206.   Mendelson, A. (1970). "On the Prevention of Addiction--A Family Agency View." G. S. Rosenthal (ed.), *The Jewish Family in a Changing World.* (pp. 149-155). Cranbury, NJ: Thomas Yoseloff.

Argues that "the concept of a 'family health maintenance program' deserves active consideration" in working to stem drug addiction.

207.   Mumey, J. (1984). *The Joy of Being Sober.* Chicago: Contemporary Books.

Argues that recovered alcoholics should get back in touch with the higher power of their church or synagogue.

208. Myerson, A. (1940). "Alcohol: A Study of Social Ambivalence." *Quarterly Journal of Studies on Alcohol, 1*(1), 13-20.

Compares the ambivalent feelings which society has toward sex with attitudes toward alcohol use. Special focus is placed on the Jewish tradition.

209. Myerson, A. (1959). "Alcoholism: The Role of Social Ambivalence." In R. G. McCarthy (ed.), *Drinking and Intoxication.* (pp. 306-312). New Haven: Yale Center of Alcohol Studies.

Adapted from Myerson (1940) "Alcohol" which appeared in the *Quarterly Journal of Studies on Alcohol 1*(1), 1-20.

210. Myerson, A. (1940). "The Social Psychology of Alcoholism." *Diseases of the Nervous System, 1*, 1-14.

Argues that neurosis and psychosis cannot be true causes of alcoholism because Jews have the same degree of these illnesses as do the general population yet they have lower alcoholism rates.

211. Novak, D. (1984). "Alcohol and Drug Abuse in the Perspective of Jewish Tradition." *Judaism, 33*(130), 220-232.

Proposes that a ban on marijuana use is consistent with Jewish tradition even though there is no ban on alcohol use.

212. Novak, D. (1985). "Alcohol and Drug Use in the Perspective of Jewish Tradition." *Halakah in a Theological Perspective.* Providence, RI: Brown University.

Investigates the question of whether there can be a halaklic ban on marijuana.

213.   Novak, D. (1986). "Alcohol and Drug Use in the Perspective of Jewish Tradition." S. J. Levy & S. B. Blume (eds.), *Addictions in the Jewish Community*. (pp. 1986). New York: Federation of Jewish Philanthropies of New York.

Reprinted from David Novak (1985) *Halakah in a Theological Tradition* Providence, RI: Brown University.

214.   Peele, S. (1983). "Is Alcoholism Different from Other Substance Abuse?" *American Psychologist, 38*(8), 963-965.

Jews would turn to eating rather than drinking when faced with emotional problems.

215.   Pittman, D. J. (1980). "An Overview of Social and Demographic Issues." M. Galanter (ed.), *Currents in Alcoholism*. 7 (pp. 341- 349). New York: Grune and Stratton.

Argues that "prohibition was a disastrous failure in a culturally pluralistic society" because different religious and ethnic groups "held radically divergent attitudes to drinking."

216.   Reiskin, H. R. (1980). *Patterns of Alcohol Usage in a Help-Seeking University: A Modified Republication of Jessor's Tri-Ethnic Study*. Boston University.

Found that Jews did not differ significantly from non-Jews in their drinking unless they were strongly attached to their ethnic heritage.

217. Riley, J. W. & Marsden, G. F. (1947). "The Medical Profession and the Problem of Alcoholism." *Quarterly Journal of Studies on Alcohol, 7*, 265-273.

Cited in Beigel and Ghertner's "Toward a Social Model."

218. Rosenman, S. (1955). "Pacts, Possessions, and the Alcoholic." *American Imago, 12*, 241-274.

Because Jews did not split their higher power into a loving-God/Satan dichotomy explains the low rate of alcoholism among Jews.

219. Rosenthal, G. S., ed. (1970). *The Jewish Family in a Changing World.* Cranbury, NJ: Thomas Yoseloff.

Includes several essays concerning alcoholism and other drug addictions.

220. Safra, Y. (12 March 1976). "B'Yahadut Artat ha B'rit Umisaviv La: Shatyanim Y'Arha B'r." *HaDoar,* 292-293.

221. Schmidt, W. & Popham, R. E. (1976). "Impressions of Jewish Alcoholism." *Journal of Studies on Alcohol, 37*(7), 931-939.

Describes the "demographic, sociocultural, and psychological characteristics, and several modes of adjustment to being Jewish alcoholics."

222. Schmidt, W. & Popham, R. E. (1980). "Impressions of Jewish Alcoholics." A. Blaine (ed.), *Alcoholism and the Jewish Community.* (pp. 153-165). New York: Federation of Jewish Philanthropies of New York.

Originally appeared in (1976) *Journal of Studies on Alcohol 37.*7, 931-939.

223.   Seller, S. C. (1985). "Alcohol Use in the Old Testament."
        Alcohol and Alcoholism, 20(1), 69-76.

        Explains that "The Old Testament offers significant lessons
        in the use and abuse of alcohol and may also contain
        pertinent clues as to why Jews, rarely abstinent, evince a
        remarkably low incidence of addictive drinking."

224.   Smith, R. (1989). "Alcoholism: Sin or Sickness?" In R. B.
        Waahlberg (ed.), *Prevention and Control/Realities and
        Aspirations, Vol. 4.* (pp. 400-406). Norway: National
        Directorate for the Prevention of Alcohol and Drug
        Problems.

        Argues that alcoholism is not a sin. Brief mention is made
        of Orthodox Jewish immigrants who eventually developed
        the same level of addiction as the people in their new
        country.

225.   Snyder, C. R. (1955). "Culture and Sobriety: A Study of
        Drinking Patterns and Sociocultural Factors Related to
        Sobriety Among Jews." *Quarterly Journal of Studies on
        Alcohol, 16*(4), 700-742.

        Focuses on the way minority status of Jews in a Gentile
        world affects their sobriety.

226.   Snyder, C. R. (1958). "Culture and Jewish Sobriety: The
        Ingroup-Outgroup Factor." In *The Jews*. Glencoe, Il: The
        Free Press.

        Investigates such factors as social pressures, intracommunity
        relationships, ethnocentrism and Jewish sobriety, religious
        ceremonies, and stereotypes.

227.   Snyder, C. R. (1962). "Culture and Jewish Sobriety: The
        Ingroup-Outgroup Factor." In D. J. Pittman & C. R. Snyder

(eds.), *Society, Culture, and Drinking Patterns.* (pp. 188-225). New York: John Wiley and Sons.

Modification of Snyder's article of the same title which appeared in Marshall Sklare (1958) *The Jews* Glencoe, IL: Free Press.

228. Snyder, C. R. & Landman, R. H. (1951). "Studies of Drinking in Jewish Culture: II: Prospectus for Sociological Research in Jewish Drinking Patterns." *Quarterly Journal of Studies on Alcohol, 12*(3), 452-474.

Summaries previous studies of Jewish drinking patterns.

229. Spiegel, M. C. "Problems of Community Denial on Recognition and Treatment of Alcoholism Among Special Ethnic Populations in Los Angeles County." *International Congress on Drugs and Alcohol.* Jerusalem.

Argues that "ethno-cultural issues need to be incorporated in any program" which target special populations.

230. Spiegel, M. C. (1986). "Profile of the Alcoholic Jew." S. J. Levy & S. B. Blume (eds.), *Addictions in the Jewish Community.* (pp. 45-61). New York: Federation of Jewish Philanthropies of New York.

Examines "the specific affects being Jewish had on the attitudes of alcoholics about their drinking, how it influences recognition of the disease and what steps they took to achieve sobriety."

231. Steinman, D. (1985). Meditations. *The JACS Journal, 2*(1), 4.

Compares the Spiritual growth of recovered alcoholics to the "counting of Omen," the 49 days leading up to *Shavuot*.

232. Straus, R. (1946). "Alcohol and the Homeless Man." *Quarterly Journal of Studies on Alcohol*, 7(3), 360-404.

Argues that "in the case of the Jews there is a reasonable explanation for their absence from the homeless ranks. As a group, Jewish people tend to take care of their own members."

233. Unkovic, C. M., Adler, R. J., & Miller, S. E. (1975). "A Contemporary Study of Jewish Alcoholism." *Alcohol Digest*, 9, vi- xiii.

234. Unkovic, C. M., Adler, R. J., & Miller, S. E. (1977). "The Contemporary State of Jewish Alcoholism." *Contemporary Jewry*, 1, 19-26.

235. Unkovic, C. M., Adler, R., & Miller, S. E. (1980). "A Contemporary Study of Jewish Alcoholism--The Significant Other Point of View." A. Blaine (ed.), *Alcoholism and the Jewish Community*. (pp. 167-185). New York: Federation of Jewish Philanthropies of New York.

Alcoholism among Jews "can be traced to such causes as: alienation, loss of religious conviction, broken homes and marriages, lack of education and poor income."

236. Wasser, A. E. (1970). "On the Prevention of Drug Abuse." G. S. Rosenthal (ed.), *The Jewish Family in a Changing World*. (pp. 145-148). Cranbury, NJ: Thomas Yoseloff.

Argues that drug abuse among Jews could best be prevented "if Jewish social agencies, synagogues, and other Jewish communal institutions made a concerted, cooperative effort to teach Jewish parents how to use 'parent power' and to strengthen the Jewish family."

237. White, H. R. (1982). "Sociological Theories of the Etiology of Alcoholism." In E. L. Gomberg, H. R. White, & J. A. Carpenter (eds.), *Alcohol, Science, and Society Revisited.* (pp. 205-232). Ann Arbor, Michigan: The University of Michigan.

Reviews studies on the incidence of alcoholism in the Jewish community.

238. Wilkinson, R. (1970). *The Prevention of Drinking Problems: Alcohol Control and Cultural Influences.* New York: Oxford University Press.

Argues that Jewish sobriety is related to cultural factors.

239. Wurzburger, W. S. (1973). "The Jewish Attitude Toward Psychedelic Religion." L. Landman (ed.), *Judaism and Drugs.* (pp. 135-143). New York: Federation of Jewish Philanthropies of New York.

Argues that "once it is recognized that mystic experience must not supersede the requirements of the *halakhic* approach, it becomes obvious that the religious ideal of the drug culture clashes head-on with the basic stance of classical rabbinic Judaism."

240. Zimberg, S. (1986). "Alcoholism Among Jews." S. J. Levy & S. B. Blume (eds.), *Addictions in the Jewish Community.* (pp. 75-85). New York: Federation of Jewish Philanthropies of New York.

Presents theories that have been used to explain the Jewish relationship to alcohol.

241. Zimberg, S. (1980). "A Socio-Psychiatric Perspective on Jewish Alcohol Abuse." A. Blaine (ed.), *Alcoholism and the Jewish Community*. (pp. 203-219). New York: Federation of Jewish Philanthropies of New York.

Offers a socio-cultural hypothesis to explain increase of Jewish alcoholics. Describes prevention plan.

242. Zimberg, S. (1977). "Sociopsychiatric Perspectives on Jewish Alcohol Abuse: Implications for the Prevention of Alcoholism." *American Journal of Drug and Alcohol Abuse*, *4*, 571-579.

Argues that the rate of alcoholism in the Jewish community increases as Jews lose their Jewish identity. Opening the doors of synagogues to AA might lessen the stigma faced by Jewish alcoholics.

243. Zimmermann, S. (1980). The Jewish Educator and the Alcoholic. A. Blaine (ed.), *Alcoholism and the Jewish Community*. (pp. 297- 303). New York: Federation of Jewish Philanthropies of New York.

Calls upon Jewish educators to spearhead a drive to educate Jews on alcoholism.

4

Comparisons to
Other Religious Groups

244. Adlaf, E. M. (1985). "Drug Use and Religious Affiliation, Feelings, and Behavior." *British Journal of Addiction*, *80*(2), 163-171.

Examines "the relationship between religious affiliation, intensity of religious feelings, frequency of church attendance on the one hand, and on the other, drug use among a sample of adolescent students."

245. Bacon, M. & Jones, M. B. (1968). *Teenage Drinking*. New York: Thomas Y. Crowell.

"The data from the teen-age studies tend to parallel the findings for adults and show again that there is some relationship between church affiliation and drinking."

246. Bacon, S. D. (1957). "Social Settings to Alcoholism: A Sociological Approach to a Medical Problem." *Journal of the American Medical Association*, *164*, 177-181.

Uses sociological data and methods to explain why different rates of alcoholism are found among different sociocultural groups. Orthodox Jews and Mormons are used throughout to illustrate his points.

247.   Beigel, A. & Ghertner, S. (1977). "Toward a Social Model: An Assessment of Social Factors Which Influence Problem Drinking and Its Treatment." B. Kissin & H. Begleiter (eds.), *Treatment and Rehabilitation of the Chronic Alcoholic.* (pp. 197-233). New York: Plenum Press.

Describes studies which show the drinking practices of Jews, Catholics, Lutherans, Episcopalians, Methodists, and Baptists.

248.   Berezin, F. G. & Roth, N. R. (1950). "Some Factors Affecting the Drinking Practices of 383 College Women in a Coeducational Institution." *Quarterly Journal of Studies on Alcohol, 11*(2), 212-221.

Found that "religious affiliation appears to be definitely associated with drinking practices. Jewish girls were found to begin their drinking at an earlier age than non-Jewish girls. Certain Protestant denominations were shown to have a lower drinking average than other Protestant groups. This may be related to the varying teaching about drinking in the respective denominations."

249.   Bock, E. W., Cochran, J. K., & Beeghley, L. (1987). "Moral Messages: The Relative Influence of Denomination on the Religiosity-Alcohol Relationship." *The Sociological Quarterly, 28*(1), 89-103.

Reference group theory is applied to the relationship between religion and alcohol use. Argues that religiosity and alcohol use is greater in proscriptive than nonproscriptive religions and that the religiosity-misuse relationship is weaker than the religiosity-use relationship.

250.   Cahalan, D. (1982). "Epidemiology: Alcohol Use in American Society." In E. L. Gomberg, H. R. White, & J. A. Carpenter (eds.), *Alcohol, Science, and Society Revisited.*

(pp. 96-118). Ann Arbor, Michigan: The University of Michigan Press.

Compares the use of alcohol between Jews, Catholics, liberal Protestants, and conservative Protestants.

251. Cahalan, D. & Cisin, I. H. (1968). "American Drinking Practices." *Quarterly Journal of Studies on Alcohol, 29,* 130-151.

Found that Jews and Episcopalians had the highest proportions of drinkers among the religious groups, but Jews also showed low proportions of heavy and escape drinkers. Although drinking was low in Protestant denominations with conservative attitudes toward drinking, the number of heavy and escape drinkers was above average among those who drank. Catholics were above average both in the number of drinkers and heavy drinkers.

252. (n.a.). (1987). *Chemical Dependency: Catholic-Jewish Reflections.* Los Angeles, California: Project Discovery.

Describes such issues as the nature of chemical dependency, historical attitudes, who is at risk, and what churches and synagogues can do about the problem.

253. Constant, G. A. (1966). "Alcoholism and the Church." *Guild of Catholic Psychiatrists Bulletin, 13*(3), 141-146.

Emphasizes that Catholics, like the Jews, need to "emphasize and re-emphasize the scientific truths about drinking" and to put into action these truths. Importance of AA stressed.

254. Cunningham, J. P. (1976). "Responsible Drinking." *NCCA Blue Book, 28,* 20-25.

Brief mention is made of wine use in the Eucharist, at Wakes, and in some Jewish rituals.

255.   Daum, M. & Lavenhar, M. A. (n.d.). *Religiosity and Drug Use: A Study of Jewish and Gentile College Students.* National Institute on Drug Abuse.

Studied relationship between religious affiliation and alcohol and other drug use.

256.   Daum, M. & Lavenhar, M. A. (1986). "Religiosity and Drug Use: A Study of Jewish and Gentile College Students." S. J. Levy & S. B. Blume (eds.), *Addictions in the Jewish Community.* (pp. 193-242). New York: Federation of Jewish Philanthropies of New York.

Originally appeared as a National Institute on Drug Abuse report.

257.   Dudley, R. L., Mutch, P. B., & Cruise, R. J. (1987). "Religious Factors and Drug Usage Among Seventh-Day Adventist Youth in North America." *Journal for the Scientific Study of Religion*, *26*(2), 218-233.

Argues that general categories such as "Catholic," "Protestant," or "Jewish" are not sufficient in attitudinal studies.

258.   Floch, M. (1947). "Imprisoned Abnormal Drinkers: Application of the Bowman-Jellinek Classification Schedule to an Institutional Sample." *Quarterly Journal of Studies on Alcohol*, *7*(4), 518-566.

Study undertaken "chiefly to discover to what extent a classification schedule of abnormal drinkers...may be of help in the understanding and treatment of abnormal drinkers committed to study, 51% were Protestants, 46%

were Roman Catholics, 5% were Greek Catholics, and 2% were Jews.

259. Goldfarb, C. (1970). "Patients Nobody Wants: Skid Row Alcoholics." *Diseases of the Nervous System, 31*, 274-281.

Study of skid row alcoholics, 60% were Catholic and 40% were Protestants. There were also three Jews, two Moslems, and one Buddhist in the total sample of 1,402.

260. Gusfield, J. R. (1963). *Symbolic Crusade: Status Politics and the American Temperance Movement*. Urbana, IL: University of Illinois Press.

Investigates the relationship between alcohol use/abuse and social/religious status. Religious affiliation and involvement in temperance are also explained.

261. Hanson, D. J. (1972). *Norm Qualities and Deviant Drinking Behavior*. Syracuse University.

Study of the different drinking rates among Jewish, Catholic, Protestant, and Mormon youth. His results were reported in his (1974) "Drinking Attitudes and Behavior Among College Students," *Journal of Alcohol and Drug Education, 19*, 6-14.

262. Hanson, D. J. (1974). "Drinking Attitudes and Behavior Among College Students." *Journal of Alcohol and Drug Education, 19*, 6-14.

Compares the drinking habits of Jewish, Catholic, Protestant, and Mormon college students.

263. Lawton, J. K. (1982). "Role of Religion: Christian Concepts." *Fourth World Congress for the Prevention of*

Alcoholism and Drug Dependency. (pp. 153-159). London: International Christian Federation.

Sets Christian attitudes toward alcohol use in the Jewish tradition.

264.   Leary, T. (1970). "The Religious Experience: Its Production and Interpretation." *Journal of Psychedelic Drugs*, *3*(1), 76-86.

Describes research which has been done to determine how LSD is used to expand religious consciousness. Jewish involvement is only briefly mentioned.

265.   Lorch, B. D. & Hughes, R. H. (1986). "Youths' Perceptions of Alcoholism." *Journal of Alcohol and Drug Education*, *31*(3), 54-63.

Surveyed youth to determine whether or not they believed alcoholism was a disease. Found that Jewish youth are least likely to consider alcoholism.

266.   Maddox, G. L. (1964). "High School Drinking Behavior: Incidental Information from Two National Surveys." *Quarterly Journal of Studies on Alcohol*, *25*(2), 339-347.

Compares the results of two surveys on high school drinking.

267.   Maghbouleh, M. D. (1979). *Psychocultural Dimension of Alcoholism, Witchcraft, Ethnic Relations, and Asceticism: A Comparative Study.* University of California at Irvine.

"Historical data on Western Christianity, Hindu-Buddhism, Judaism, and Confucianism were examined to determine their predominant cultural schema for the reconciliation of opposites and the degree to which each group employed its respective schemas in justifying asceticism, inquisition, witchhunts, ethnic warfare (e.g. crusades, genocide), and prohibition or religious abstinence from alcohol."

268. Mulford, H. A. (1964). "Drinking and Deviant Behavior, USA 1963." *Quarterly Journal of Studies on Alcohol, 25,* 634-650.

Methodists, Baptists, and Jews were found to have the lowest rates of heavy drinking.

269. Popham, R. E. (1955). "A Statistical Report Relating to Alcoholism and the Use of Alcohol Beverages in Canada." *International Journal of the Addictions, 1,* 5-22.

Compares differences between users and abstainers of alcohol between Canadians and Americans. Information is provided on use by Jews, Catholics, and Protestants.

270. Popham, R. E. (1959). "Canada." R. G. McCarthy (ed.), *Drinking and Intoxication.* (pp. 170-174). New Haven, CT: College and University Press.

Taken from (1955) "Statistical Report Relating to Alcoholism and the Use of Alcoholic Beverages in Canada" *International Journal of the Addictions, 1,* 5-22.

271. Proctor, R. C. (1984). "History of Drinking in America." *Southern Medical Journal, 77*(7), 886-892.

A history of drinking in America which focuses not only on attitudes toward alcohol use, but also on attitudes toward excessive drinking. Gives statistics on the percentage of Catholics, Protestants, and Jews who drink.

272.   Riley, J. W. & Marder, C. F. (1947). "The Social Pattern of Alcoholic Drinking." *Quarterly Journal of Studies on Alcohol, 8,* 265-273.

Found that 59% of the Protestants, 79% of the Catholics, and 87% of the Jews drank.

273.   Robins, L. N. & Smith, E. M. (1980). "Longitudinal Studies of Alcohol and Drug Problems: Sex Differences." O. J. Kalant (ed.), *Alcohol and Drug Problems in Women.* (pp. 203-232). New York: Plenum Press.

Summarizes research which shows that Catholics drink more than Protestants and Jews.

274.   Skolnick, J. (1958). "Religious Affiliation and Drinking Behavior." *Quarterly Journal of Studies on Alcohol, 19*(3), 452-470.

Reports the findings of a survey among Jewish, Methodist, and Episcopalian college students who drink. Religious affiliation significantly influenced drinking behavior more than did regional background, social class position, maturity, and religious participation.

275.   Smart, R. & Fejer, D. (1969). "Illicit LSD Users: Their Social Backgrounds, Drug Use and Psychopathology." *Journal of Health and Social Behavior, 10*(4), 297-308.

Found there was a significant difference between LSD users and non-users in how they practiced their religion. Most of the LSD users who have regularly attended church were followers of Zen Buddhism. Of the sample studied 18% of the users were Jewish.

276.   Snyder, C. R. (1955). "Culture and Sobriety: A Study of Drinking Patterns and Sociocultural Factors Related to

Sobriety Among Jews." *Quarterly Journal of Studies on Alcohol, 16*(1), 101- 177.

Compares drinking practices of Jews to British Protestants and Irish Catholics and differences of drinking practices between Orthodox, Conservative, Reformed, and Secular Jews. Based on Snyder's dissertation.

277. Stivers, R. (1983). "Religion and Alcoholism." B. Kissin & H. Begleiter (eds.), *The Pathogenesis of Alcoholism.* (pp. 341-364). New York: Plenum Press.

Compares Catholic Irish-American and Jewish drinking patterns and rates of alcoholism.

278. Waring, M. L., Petraglia, G. & Busby, E. (1984). Drinking Patterns of Graduate Social Work Students. *Journal of Alcohol and Drug Education, 29*(3), 9-18.

Study of the drinking habits of social work students in which 14% of the students were Protestant, 15% were Jewish, 57% were Catholic, and 14% stated no religion.

279. Wechsler, H., Demone, H. W., Thum, D., & Kasey, E. (1970). "Religious-Ethnic Differences in Alcohol Consumption." *Journal of Health and Social Behavior, 11*(1), 21-29.

Data collected on 8,461 patients admitted to an emergency room. Found that "the proportion of patients with positive indications of alcohol was lowest among Jewish persons and Italian Catholics. High frequencies were found for Irish, Canadian, and native born Catholics, as well as native born Protestants."

5

Comparisons to
Other Cultural Groups

280. (1989). "You Gotta Have Hope." *The Catholic World, 232* (1390), 158-163.

An interview with Dr. Robert F. Stuckey. Topics covered include family dynamics, intervention, AA, Al-Anon, and accepting a higher power in recovery. Brief mention is made of the low rate of alcoholism in Israel, China, and Southern Italy because the family structure in those places is seen to control individuals.

281. Bales, R. F. (1944). *The "Fixation Factor" in Alcohol Addiction: An Hypothesis Derived from a Comparative Study of Irish and Jewish Social Norms.* Cambridge, MA: Harvard University.

Compares Irish and Jewish drinking patterns.

282. Bandel, R. (17 April 1920). *Zeitschrift fur Hygiene und Intektionskrankseiten,* 259+.

"His examination of the mortality data of married and unmarried men in Bavaria, Berlin, and Budapest and of Jewish people and Gentiles comparatively in Prussia, Berlin, and Budapest again convinces him that when the consumption of alcohol was greatly reduced during the war or through racial habits of temperance, the death rate was also low." [cited in Edwin Kopf (1932) "Review of Recent Literature on Alcohol as a Community Health Problem." *Alcohol and Man*, Haven Emerson, (ed.) New York: MacMillan.]

283. Becker, R. (1932). "Die Geisteserkrankungen Bei Den Juden in Polen." *Allg. Z. Psychiat*, *96*, 47-66.

284. Bell, P. (1984). "Anthropological Overview of Substance Abuse: A Social Policy Prevention Approach." *Alabama Journal of Medical Sciences*, *21*(2), 162-165.

   Explores alcohol and drug use from an anthropological and socio-cultural view. Special attention is given to blacks, native Americans, and Jews.

285. Boscarino, J. (1980). "Isolating the Effects of Ethnicity on Drinking Behavior: A Multiple Classification Analysis of Barroom Attendance." *Addictive Behaviors*, *5*, 307-312.

   Studies Irish-Americans, English Americans, Italian-Americans, and Jewish Americans. Argues that more demographic variables need to be used in studies of ethnic drinking patterns.

286. Cahalan, D. (1970). *Problem Drinkers: A National Survey*. San Francisco: Jossey-Bass.

   Compares Jewish drinking practices to the practices of people from other cultures.

287. Casselman, J. (1983). "Frontieres Socioculturelles." *Alcool au Sante: Alcoolisation Phenomene Sans Frontieres*. (pp. 20-23). Paris: np.

Mention is made that Jewish immigrants to the United States preserve the drinking habits of their country of origin. The text is in French.

288.	Caution, G. (1982). *Ethnic Drinking Patterns*. Orangeburg, SC: South Carolina State College.

Reviews existing research literature on alcohol consumption of Jews, blacks, and native Americans.

289.	Chafetz, M. E. (1964). "Consumption of Alcohol in the Far and Middle East." *New England Journal of Medicine, 271*, 297-301.

Investigates the rate of alcoholism, social attitudes toward alcoholism, and how alcoholics are treated.

290.	Cisin, I. H. (1978). "Formal and Informal Social Controls Over Drinking." J. A. Ewing & B. A. Rouse (eds.), *Drinking*. (pp. 145-158). Chicago: Nelson-Hall.

Cites the low rate of alcoholism among Jews and Italians even though both cultural groups drink heavily.

291.	Eckhardt, W. (1967). "Alcoholic Values and Alcoholics Anonymous." *Quarterly Journal of Studies on Alcohol, 28*(2), 277-288.

Studied the twelve longest case histories which appeared in *Alcoholics Anonymous*. Briefly mentions cultural values which influence Jewish and Irish drinking patterns.

292.	Eddy, R. (1887). *Alcohol in History, an Account of Intemperance in all Ages; Together With a History of the*

Various Methods Employed for Its Removal. New York: National Temperance Society and Publication House.

Study of drinking in various cultures.

293. Faris, R. E. & Dunham, H. W. (1939). *Mental Disorders in Urban Areas.* Chicago: University of Chicago Press.

The low rate of alcoholism in two of the communities which were studied was attributed to the high percent of Russian Jews living in those areas.

294. Freund, P. J. (1980). "Armenian-American Drinking Patterns: Ethnicity, Family, and Religion." *Alcoholism: Journal of Alcoholism and Related Addictions, 16*(1-2), 9-25.

Compares the drinking patterns of Jews and Armenian-Americans, both of which the author claims have low rates of alcoholism.

295. Glad, D. D. (1947). "Attitudes and Experiences of American- Jewish and American-Irish Male Youths as Related to Differences in Adult Rates of Inebriety." *Quarterly Journal of Studies on Alcohol, 8*(3), 406-472.

Revised version of authors dissertation. Investigates the differences between Jewish-American and Irish-American drinking practices.

296. Glad, D. D. (1947). *Attitudes and Experiences of American-Jewish and American-Irish Male Youths as Related to Differences in Inebriety Rates.* Sanford, CA: Stanford, University.

A revised version of the dissertation was published under the same title in (1947) *Quarterly Journal of Studies on Alcohol 8*,3: 406-472.

297.   Gomez, J. (1984). "Learning to Drink: The Influence of Impaired Psychosocial Development." *Journal of Psychosomatic Research, 28*(5), 403-410.

Recommends that "a cultural shift towards the Jewish or Italian view of drinking would be of immense value, propagated by those in charge of their own children: with alcohol introduced early and naturally, not as a manly treat, and excess regarded as childish and unacceptable."

298.   Goodwin, D.W. (1979). "Protective Factors in Alcoholism." *Drug and Alcohol Dependence, 4*, 99-100.

Cites evidence that more Jews than non-Jews have a psychological protection against heavy drinking.

299.   Greeley, A. M. & McCready, W. C. (1978). "A Preliminary Reconnaissance Into the Persistence and Explanation of the Ethnic Subculture Drinking Patterns." *Medical Anthropology, 2*(4), 31-51.

Presents "socialization" model which accounts for much of the cultural differences among white ethnic groups in the United States.

300.   Greeley, A., McCreedy, W. & Thiesen, G. (1980). *Ethnic Drinking Subcultures*. New York: Praeger Publishers.

Information on alcohol use and abuse in the Jewish community is found throughout.

301. Haberman, P. W. (1970). "Denial of Drinking in a Household Survey." *Quarterly Journal of Studies on Alcohol, 31*(3), 710-717.

"About one-third of a representative sample of New Yorkers denied drinking alcoholic beverages, a proportion considerably larger than that found in national surveys. More denial of drinking was found among older than younger respondents, the less-educated, Puerto Ricans, Italians, and Jews. It is suggested that younger Italians and Jews are not following traditional drinking patterns and that the older ones misinterpreted the question."

302. Haberman, P. W. & Sheinberg, J. (1967). "Implicative Drinking Reported in a Household Survey: A Corroborative Note on Subgroup Differences." *Quarterly Journal of Studies on Alcohol, 28*(3), 538-543.

Italians and Jews were found to be the least vulnerable groups for alcoholism.

303. Heath, D. B. (1982). "In Other Cultures, They Also Drink." E. L. Gomberg & et al. (eds.), *Alcohol, Science, and Society Revisited*. (pp. 63-79). Ann Arbor: University of Michigan Press.

Describes the variety of cross-cultural studies which have been used to study drinking patterns.

304. Heath, D. B. (1984). "Cross-Cultural Studies of Alcohol Use." M. Glanter (ed.), *Recent Developments in Alcoholism*. (2). (pp. 405-415). New York: Plenum Press.

Describes the variety of cross-cultural studies which have been used to study drinking patterns.

305.	Heath, D. (1987). "A Decade of Development in the Anthropological Study of Alcohol Use, 1970-1980." In M. Douglas (ed.), *Constructive Drinking.* (pp. 16-69). Cambridge, Massachusetts: Cambridge University Press.

Summarizes literature on Jewish alcoholics.

306.	Heath, D. B. (1983). "Etiologic Aspects of Alcohol and Drug Abuse." In E. Gottheil (eds.), *Etiologic Aspects of Alcohol and Drug Abuse.* (pp. 223-237). Springfield, Illinois: Charles C. Thomas.

Includes a section in which he summarizes some theories on Jewish alcoholism.

307.	Heath, D. B. (1982). "Sociocultural Variants in Alcoholism." E. M. Pattison & E. Kaufman (eds.), *Encyclopedic Handbook of Alcoholism.* (pp. 426-440). New York: Gardner Press.

Mention is made of the low rate of alcoholism among Jews.

308.	Hill, T. M. (1977). "Survey of Jewish Drinking Patterns." *Military Chaplain's Review*, 65-77.

Surveys genetic, environmental, physiological, psychological, and sociological factors relating to alcoholism among Jews, as well as education, strategies and treatment for non-Jews as well as Jews.

309.	Kandel, D. B., Adler, I., & Sudit, M. (1981). "The Epidemiology of Adolescent Drug Use in France and Israel." *American Journal of Public Health*, *71*(3), 256-265.

Study of alcohol and other drug use (including tobacco) of youth in France and Israel. Affects of religiosity on rate of use was one factor studied.

310. Kandel, D. B. & Sudit, M. (1982). "Drinking Practices Among Urban Adults in Israel, Cross-Cultural Comparison." *Quarterly Journal of Studies on Alcohol*, 43(1), 1-16.

Compares the rates of alcoholism in American and Israel. Emphasis on use of wine in Jewish religious rituals.

311. King, A. R. (1961). "The Alcohol Problem in Israel." *Quarterly Journal of Studies on Alcohol*, 22(2), 321-324.

Gives cultural factors and social-solidarity issues to explain the low rate of alcoholism among Israelis.

312. Kissin, B. (1977). "Theory and Practice in the Treatment of Alcoholism." B. Kissin & H. Begleiter (eds.), *Treatment and Rehabilitation of the Chronic Alcoholic.* (pp. 1-51). New York: Plenum Press.

Cites a study which shows that Jewish alcoholics have more psychopathology than Irish alcoholics.

313. Kissin, B. & Hanson, M. (1982). "Bio-psyco-social Perspective in Alcoholism." J. Solomon (ed.), *Alcoholism and Clinical Psychiatry.* (pp. 1-19). New York: Plenum Medical Book.

Argues that "Jewish alcoholics might be more "psychologically vulnerable" to alcohol than alcoholics from other ethnic groups.

314. Knupfer, G. & Room, R. (1967). "Drinking Patterns and Attitudes of Irish, Jewish and White Protestant American Men." *Quarterly Journal of Studies on Alcohol*, 28(4), 676-699.

Compares drinking practices among the Irish, Jews, and Protestants in the San Francisco Bay area.

315. Lemert, E. M. (1956). "Alcoholism: Theory, Problem, and Challenge III: Alcoholism and the Sociocultural Situation." *Quarterly Journal of Studies on Alcohol, 17*(2), 306-317.

Proposes that Jewish sobriety is related to ritual use of alcohol. Finds this theory consistent with studies done on costal plains Indians.

316. Letman, S. T. & Edwards, D. W. (1982). *Alcoholism in the Urban Community*. Chicago: Loyola University.

Includes a chapter on "Irish and Jewish Drinking Patterns, and the Black American." Focuses on environmental factors leading to rates of alcoholism.

317. Madden, J. S. (1982). "Some Cultural Aspects of Drinking." *British Journal on Alcohol and Alcoholism, 17*(1), 1-4.

Citing the Chinese and Jews as examples, the author argues that it is possible to decrease the number of alcohol problems without resorting to prohibition.

318. Martin, P. R. (1981). "Human Genetics of Alcoholism." *Substance and Alcohol Actions/Misuse, 2*(5/6), 389-406.

Mention is made that Jews, more than non-Jews seem to have a "protective" alcohol-induced dysphoria.

319. McCready, W. C., Greeley, A. M., & Thiesen, G. (1983). "Ethnicity and Nationality in Alcoholism." In Kissin Benjamin & H. Begleiter (eds.), *The Pathogenesis of Alcoholism*. (6). New York: Plenum Press.

Compares the drinking patterns of Irish Catholics, Italian Americans, Jews, and Swedes.

320. McKirkan, D. J. & Peterson, P. L. (1989). "Psychological and Cultural Factors in Alcohol and Drug Abuse: An Analysis of a Homosexual Community." *Addictive Behaviors, 14,* 555-563.

Argued that while some cultures, such as the Jewish, have socialization practices which make their members resistant to substance abuse, "the urban homosexual culture may be a clear example of the opposite."

321. McVernon, J. (1987). "Addictions: A National Priority." *NCCA Blue Book, 39,* 39-46.

Examples used to show how drugs are used in various cultures include the use of wine during Christian liturgy and at the Jewish Seder.

322. Meyer, A. (1932). "Alcohol as a Psychiatric Problem." H. Emerson (ed.), *Alcohol and Man.* (pp. 273-309). New York: MacMilliam.

Compares the percentage of alcoholic cases to the total number of patients suffering psychosis who were admitted into a state hospital, Found that there were fewer cases of alcoholic Jews.

323. Plaut, T. F. A., ed. (1967). *Alcohol Problems: A Report to the Nation by the Cooperative Commission on the Study of Alcoholism.* New York: Oxford University Press.

Explains that low rates of alcoholism are found in Italian-American and Jewish-American families because these groups make clear distinctions between acceptable and unacceptable drinking and introduce youth to alcohol at an early age.

324. Rawat, A. K. (1983). "Genetic Aspects of Ethanol Disposition and Dependence." *Neurobehavioral Toxicology and Teratology, 5*(2), 193-199.

Brief description of Jewish drinking patterns.

325. Roberts, B. H. & Myers, J. K. (1967). "Religion, National Origin, Immigration, and Mental Illness." S. I. Weinberg (ed.), *Sociology and Mental Disorders.* (pp. 68-72). Chicago: Aldine.

Concludes that alcoholism was highest in Irish-Catholics and "psychoneurotic disorders were more frequent among Jews."

326. Robins, L. N., Bates, W. M., & O'Neal, P. (1962). "Adult Drinking Patterns of Former Problem Children." D. J. Pittman & C. R. Snyder (eds.), *Society, Culture, and Drinking.* (pp. 395-412). New York: Wiley.

Of the Jews in the study, 20% were considered alcoholic and 20% were considered heavy drinkers. Aspects of childhood which differentiated alcoholics from non-alcoholics were "the social status of the family, the adequacy of the parents, and the number of antisocial symptoms."

327. Sargent, M. J. (1969). *A Cross Cultural Study of Drinking Behavior and Attitudes of Australian, Jewish, Chinese, and Japanese People.* University of New South Wales.

Compared the drinking practices and attitudes of Australians, Jews, Chinese, and Japanese college students. Jewish group included more moderate and fewer light drinkers than she had predicted. Summarized in Sargent (1971) "A Cross-Cultural Study of Attitudes and Behavior Towards Alcohol and Drugs," *British Journal of Sociology, 22,* 83-96.

328. Sargent, M. J. (1971). "A Cross-Cultural Study of Attitudes and Behavior Towards Alcohol and Drugs." *British Journal of Sociology, 22,* 83-96.

Found that contrary to what she predicted, the Jewish group included more moderate and fewer light drinkers than expected. Other groups investigated were Australians, Japanese, and Chinese.

329. Shalloo, J. P. (1941). "Some Cultural Factors in the Etiology of Alcoholism." *Quarterly Journal of Studies on Alcohol, 2*(3), 464-478.

Attention is placed on alcohol use during religious festivals.

330. Staski, E. (1983). *Alcohol Consumption Among Irish-Americans and Contributions from Archeology.* University of Arizona at Tucson.

Found that no correlation exists, at least for household consumption, between Jewish-American and Irish-American drinkers.

331. Ullman, A. D. (1960). "Ethnic Differences in the First Drinking Experience." *Social Problems, 8*(1), 45-56.

Groups with high rates of alcoholism permit their members to be introduced to alcohol by non-family members. Jews were one group studied.

332. Westermeyer, J. (1982). "Alcoholism and Services for Ethnic Populations." E. M. Pattison & E. Kaufman (eds.), *Encyclopedic Handbook of Alcoholism.* (pp. 709-717). New York: Gardner Press.

Describes the variations of alcohol use in various cultures. Jews are mentioned.   Identical to his "Alcoholism and Psychiatry."

333.   Westermeyer, J. (1982). "Alcoholism and Psychiatry: A Cross- Cultural Perspective." J. Solomon (ed.), *Alcoholism and Cultural Psychiatry*. (pp. 35-47). New York: Plenum Medical Book Company.

Describes the variations of alcohol use in several cultures. Jews are mentioned.   Identical to his "Alcoholism and Services for Ethnic Populations."

334.   Williams, R. J. (1947). "The Etiology of Alcoholism: A Working Hypothesis Involving the Interplay of Heredity and Environmental Factors." *Quarterly Journal of Studies on Alcohol*, 7(4), 567-587.

Emphasis on Jewish and Irish alcoholics.

6

First Person Stories and Case Studies

335. (n.a.). (1986). "Author of 'Hatikavah' Died of Alcoholism. *The JACS Journal*, *3*(2), 6.

A case study of Naphtali Herz.

336. Bahr, H. M. (1973). *Skid Row: An Introduction to Disaffiliation*. New York: Oxford University Press.

Includes a case study of a Jewish woman on skid row.

337. Berkovits, E. (1973). "Instant Mysticism and Chemical Religion." L. Landman (ed.), *Judaism and Drugs*. (pp. 97-133). New York: Federation of Jewish Philanthropies of New York.

Analyzes the mystical experiences caused by hallucinogenic drugs.

338. Blume, S. B. (1986). "Studying Alcohol Problems in Jewish People: A Memoir." S. J. Levy & S. B. Blume (eds.), *Addictions in the Jewish Community*. (pp. 93-100). New York: Federation of Jewish Philanthropies of New York.

Explains why author studies Jewish alcoholics.

339.   Catherine H. (1989). *Talking to a Higher Power*. Park Ridge, Illinois: Parkside Publishing Co.

Cites the experience of a Jewish woman.

340.   Cohen, A. B. [pseud]. (November 1981). "Wanted Help for Orthodox Addicts." *Jewish Observer*, 9-13.

Story of addiction and recovery through Pills Anonymous. AA is mentioned.

341.   Courtwright, D., Joseph, H., & Des Jarlais, D. (1989). *Addicts Who Survived: An Oral History of Narcotic Use In America, 1923-1965*. Knoxville, Tennessee: University of Tennessee Press.

Information is provided on drug trafficking and narcotic use by Jews.

342.   Fulman, R. (10 June 1977). "Jews and Alcoholism." *New York Daily News*.

Includes a case study of a Jewish, female alcoholic.

343.   G.N.G. (April, 1967). "My Son, the Alcoholic." *Box 1980* [The Grapevine], 2.

Argues against myth that there are few Jewish alcoholics.

344.   Greenfield, F. (1988). Pieces of Freddie Greenfield: Dickie's Word Against Anybody's. *Fag Rag*, *44*, 20.

Claims that an advantage of being a gay, Jewish addict in New York City "is that there are a lot of other jewish (sic) dope fiends nearer my age."

345.   Gringras, N. "Out of the Depths." unpublished manuscript.

Shares experience of celebrating high holidays with Jewish alcoholics in treatment.

346. J.H. (1987). "How It Was." *Box 1980* [The Grapevine], *44*(3), 36.

Mentions that his 30 year association with AA has helped change his hatred of homosexuals, Jews, and blacks.

347. Jacobson, M. (1980). "A Nice Jewish Girl Like Me Became an Alcoholic." A. Blaine (ed.), *Alcoholism and the Jewish Community.* (pp. 327-331). New York: Federation of Jewish Philanthropies of New York.

Tells the story of her addiction and recovery from alcoholism.

348. Kenny, K. (1988). *It Only Hurts When I Grow Up: Stories from Covenant House for Hurting Kids.* New York, New York: Paulist Press.

Includes case study of Morey, a Jewish drug addict who was helped by Covenant House.

349. Kimball, C. (1905). "Amusements and Social Life: Philadelphia." C. S. Bernheimer (ed.), *The Russian Jew in the United States.* (pp. 233-248). Philadelphia: John C. Winston.

Includes a case study of a drunken young man at a dance to demonstrate the problems which some young Jews have in adapting to the freedom they now enjoy since leaving Russia.

350. Manners, C.P. (13 February 1981). "I Was An Amateur Lush." *Baltimore Jewish News, 40,* 42-43.

Tells of her addiction to alcohol and her spontaneous recovery.

351. Michael K. (1990) "Twice Chosen." *Jacs Journal*, 7(1), 6.

Explains why he was chosen by his higher power to be an addict.

352. (n.a.). (1989). "Not Necessarily The Jews." *JACS Journal*, 6(1), 4-5.

Reports on the case of John Norfolk, an atheist who claimed his constitutional rights were violated when he was forced to attend AA.

353. Pfefferman, N. (1988). "Coming to Terms with Alcoholism." *The Jewish Journal*, 2(42), 4.

Uses case studies to show how some Jewish alcoholics avoid drinking during the December holidays.

354. Pfefferman, N. (1988). "One Man's Story." *The Jewish Journal*, 2(42), 4.

Tells of Philip Sigal's alcoholism and recovery.

355. Roth, L. (1959). *Beyond My Worth*. New York: Popular Library.

Describes early years of author's during which she converted from Judaism to Catholicism.

356. Roth, L. (1954). *I'll Cry Tomorrow*. New York: Frederick Fell, Inc.

Autobiography of Jewish alcoholic who recovered through AA.

357. Selvig, D. & Riley, D. (1980). *High and Dry*. New York: Pinnacle Books.

Cites cases of treating alcoholic priests, rabbis, and Jewish businessmen.

358. Siegel-Itzkovich, J. (January 1989). Alcoholic Rehabilitation. *Jerusalem Post*, 5.

Describes work of Pnina Eldar, director of the Israel Society for the Prevention of Alcoholism.

359. Spiegel, M. C. (1982). "Hard Drinking." *Present Tense*, 9(2), 14-17.

Uses case studies to counter the idea that Jews cannot be alcoholic.

360. Spiegel, M. C. (Summer, 1988). "The Last Taboo: Dare We Speak About Incest." *Lilith*, 10-12.

Cites Jewish male alcoholic and Jewish male cocaine abusers as examples of incest purveyors.

361. Spiegel, M. C. (July 22-July 28, 1988). "The Last Taboo: Dare We Speak About Incest?" *The Jewish Journal*, 18,23.

Reprinted from (Summer, 1988) *Lilith*, 10-12.

362. Stevens, C. (1989). "My Stepfather Is an Alcoholic." In E. N. Hayes (ed.), *Adult Children of Alcoholics Remember*. (pp. 130- 142). New York, New York: Harmony Books.

Jewish adult child of an alcoholic describes her family experience and her own heavy drinking and drug use is also described.

363. Sullivan, E., Bissell, L., & Williams, E. (1988). *Chemical Dependency in Nursing.* Menco Park: Addison-Wesley.

Need for treatment providers to be sensitive to the religious needs of clients. Example of an orthodox Jewish man is used.

364. Tilleraas, P. (1990). *Circle of Hope: Our Stories of AIDS, Addiction, and Recovery.* Center City, MN: Hazelden.

Includes case study of Lewis, a gay, recovered alcoholic whose maternal grandparents were Russian Jews.

365. (n.a.). (1983). "To Keep From Being Controlled: An Interview with Misha Cohen." In J. Swallow, *Out From Under.* (pp. 71-78). San Francisco: Spinsters Ink.

Explains how acupuncture can be used in detox. Chinese meditation, natural healing, and the political ramifications of recovery are also mentioned.

366. Washton, A. M., Zahm, D. L., & Gold, M. S. (1986). "Cocaine and Jews." S. J. Levy & S. B. Blume (eds.), *Addictions in the Jewish Community.* (pp. 161-179). New York: Federation of Jewish Philanthropies of New York.

Three case studies are presented.

367. Weinstein, S. (April 4 - April 10, 1988). "Jews and Alcoholism: Destroying the Old-Age Myth of Immunity." *Jewish Journal,* 9-10.

Uses case studies to demonstrate the problem of alcoholism in the Jewish community.

7

Jewish Involvement
in Alcoholics Anonymous

368. (n.a.). (August, 1969). "After the Fall." *Box 1980* [The Grapevine], 17-19.

Tells story of a Jewish alcoholic's addiction, relapse, and recovery through AA.

369. (n.a.). (1985). "After the Fall." *Best of the Grapevine.* (pp. 168-171). New York: AA World Services.

Reprinted from the August 1969 issue of Box 1980.

370. Bayer, E. & Levy, S. J. (1980). Notes on the First Retreat for Jewish Alcoholics. A. Blaine (ed.), *Alcoholism and the Jewish Community.* (pp. 333-345). New York: Federation of Jewish Philanthropies of New York.

Description of the first retreat held for Jewish alcoholics who had recovered through AA.

371. Bebe L. (1986). "The Princess and the Priest." *The JACS Journal*, *3*(2), 4-5.

Testimonial on the difficulty the author faced as a Jew trying to come to a higher power in AA. Emphasizes the need for spiritual materials to be published in the Jewish tradition.

372.   Berg, S. L. (1989). *AA, Spiritual Issues, and the Treatment of Lesbian and Gay Alcoholics.* East Lansing, Michigan: Michigan State University.

Compares negative reaction some lesbians and gays and some Jews have to the Christian nature of AA.

373.   Berman, S. (1988). *The Twelve Steps and Jewish Tradition.* Center City: Hazelden.

An AA alcoholic helps other Jews come to terms with the AA program.

374.   C.G. (April, 1990). Stand and Be Counted. *Box 1980* [The Grapevine], *46*(11), 40.

Talks about separating Judaism from alcoholism as issues in recovery.

375.   Carol H. (1989). Letter. *JACS Journal, 6*(1), 7.

She is frequently the only Jew in AA.

376.   Chambers, F. T. (1953). "Analysis and Comparison of Three Treatment Measures for Alcoholism: Antabuse, the Alcoholics Anonymous Approach, and Psychotherapy." *British Journal of Addiction, 50,* 29-41.

377.   Cohen, A. B. [pseud]. (Winter 1982). "New Help for Jewish Addicts." *Jewish Action.*

An AA was formed by Orthodox Jews.

378. Davis, E. B. (n.d.). *The New Way of Life*. Cleveland, OH: Alcoholics Anonymous.

    Describing the A.A. way of life. Emphasizes that any higher power is acceptable.

379. (n.a.). (1976). *Do You Think You're Different?* New York, New York: Alcoholics Anonymous World Services, Inc.

    Includes the story of a Jewish alcoholic who recovered through AA.

380. Flores, P. (1988). "Alcoholics Anonymous: A Phenomenological and Existential Perspective." *Alcoholism Treatment Quarterly*, *5*(1), 73-94.

    Compares AA to existential philosophy and to phenomenology. Emphasis on shame, suffering, and narcissism. Notes the similarities between Victor Frankl's understanding of suffering in a concentration camp with how AA alcoholics understand suffering.

381. (n.a.). (April 1952). "From Priest to Preacher." *Box 1980* [The Grapevine], 5-7.

    Mentions that the welcome extended "by social parlor, parish house and synagogue to AA groups has provided the rooms where many an alcoholic has found" sobriety.

382. Glass, C. (1985). "The Twelve Steps and the Jewish Tradition." *JACS Journal*, *2*(1), 6-8,12.

    Explains how AA's twelve steps are consistent with Jewish theology.

383. Gringras, N. (1984). "Judaism, Addiction, and Faith: The Spiritual Odyssey of Recovery." *JACS Journal*, *1*(2), 3.

Explains how the AA program compliments the Jewish spiritual tradition.

384.   Gringras, N. (Winter 1984). "Judaism, Addiction, and Faith: The Spiritual Odyssey of Recovery." *JACS Journal*, 9-11.

Explains how the AA program helps alcoholics to overcome denial, shame, and despair.

385.   Gringras, N. (1986). "Judaism, Addiction and Faith: The Spiritual Odyssey of Recovery." S. J. Levy & S. B. Blume (eds.), *Addictions in the Jewish Community*. (pp. 265-296). New York: Federation of Jewish Philanthropies of New York.

Presents a Jewish interpretation of alcoholism and recovery through AA.

386.   J. (1987). AA in Israel. *JACS Newsletter*, 4(1), 5-6.

Describes AA meetings he attended in Israel.

387.   Jim G. (1990) "Not Mysticism." *JACS Journal*, 7(1), 4-5.

A rabbi explains how Jewish mysticism can be applied to the AA program.

388.   L.S. (May 1977). Lost and Found *Box 1980* [The Grapevine], 21.

Shares experience of recovery in AA.

389.   Larry G. (1989). A Meeting in Israel. *JACS Journal*, 6(1), 5-6.

Tells about his spiritual development and ability to combine a study of Judaism with his AA program.

390. Master, L. (1989). "Jewish Experiences of Alcoholics Anonymous." *Smith College Studies in Social Work, 59*(2), 183-199.

391. Miller, J. (1987). Reflections on the Lord's Prayer. *JACS Journal, 4*(1), 9.

   Expresses concern about people who encourage Jews not to say the Lord's Prayer at the end of AA, NA, and Al-Anon meetings because of its association with Christianity. Fears that such "encouragement" might keep Jews away from meetings that save Jewish lives.

392. (n.a.). (September, 1956). "The Mingled Dust." *Box 1980* [The Grapevine], 39.

   Reports on Jewish legend concerning the creation of man.

393. (n.a.). (1988). More Alike Than Different. *Box 1980* [The Grapevine], *45*(7), 2-3.

   Jewish author tells about attending AA meetings in Israel.

394. Robertson, N. (21 February 1988). "The Changing World of Alcoholics Anonymous." *New York Times Magazine*, 40.

   Summarized from (1988) *Getting Better* New York: William Morrow.

395. Robertson, N. (1988). *Getting Better: The Story of Alcoholics Anonymous*. New York: William Morrow.

   Author's experience in AA. Jewish issues are mentioned throughout.

396. Rothberg, S. A. (1986). "Hitting the Kneel on the Head." *The JACS Journal, 3*(2), 7.

Argues that "kneeling is not only a matter of physical posture, it can be a spiritual attitude." Thus, Jews can kneel while standing up.

397.   Rothberg, S. A. (1989). "Hitting the Kneel on the Head." S. L. Berg (ed.), *Alcoholism and Pastoral Ministry.* (pp. 122). Lake Orion, MI: Guest House.

Reprinted from (1986) *JACS Journal, 3*(2), 7.

398.   Spiegel, M. C. (October 1986). "Shabbat Shuvah: A Time for Turning." *Jewish Advocate*, 10.

Relates the twelve steps of recovery to the celebration of *Shabbat Shuvah*. Shows how the philosophy behind twelve step programs merges with Judaism.

399.   Steinberg, P. (September 6-12, 1990). "Secret Revealed: 'Jewish Denial' Holds Back Treatment for Drug Addiction." *Jewish Journal*.

Describes issue of denial within the Jewish community and the founding of the Exodus Center.

400.   Steinman, D. (Winter 1984). "Judaism and the Twelve Steps." *JACS Journal*, 6.

Argues that "while the Steps are not derived from Jewish sources, they do parallel basic Jewish concepts."

401.   Swartz, M. B. (1987). "An Unusual Encounter with AA." *JACS Journal, 4*(1), 8-9.

Compares the English and Hebrew AA meetings he attended in Israel.

402. Twerski, A. J. (1986). "Judaism and the Twelve Steps." S. J. Levy & S. B. Blume (eds.), *Addictions in the Jewish Community.* (pp. 123-133). New York: Federation of Jewish Philanthropies of New York.

Offers a Jewish interpretation of AA's Twelve Steps.

403. Twerski, A. J. (1986). "Spirituality, Prayer, the Twelve Steps, and Judaism." *JACS Journal*, *3*(1), 6-9.

Argues that the Christian nature of AA is not inherent in AA and that Jewish theologians need to develop literature for recovering Jews. Gives a Jewish interpretation of the twelve steps.

404. Winner, J. (1988). "On Discrimination and Intolerance." *Save Our Selves*, *1*(3), 1.

Argues that he is disturbed by the "demeaning and erroneous portrayal of the nonbeliever." Examples are cited from AA literature and brief mention is made of Jews.

8

Jewish Alcoholics, Chemically Dependent Persons, and Significant Others (JACS)

405. Calarino, M. (1983) "Fighting Alcoholism." *Present Tense*, 9(3), 3-4.

Letter which describes nature of JACS.

406. David. "Address." [Southeastern Conference on Alcoholism and Drug Abuse]. Atlanta, GA.

David describes the history of JACS and its current mission.

407. (n.a.). "The Issues Addressed." *JACS Journal*, 7(1), 4.

Four letters written to JACS office addressing such issues as AA, the Lord's prayer, retreats, and JACS.

408. (n.a.). (n.d.). *JACS*.

Describes what JACS is and what it is not.

409. (n.a.). (n.d.). *The JACS Foundation*. (np).

Describes the structure of the JACS Foundation.

410. (n.a.). (March 25, 1990) *Jewish Spirituality and Recovery.* (np).

Program for retreat sponsored by JACS.

411. Kaplan, D. (1987). "Some Thoughts on Jewish Prayer and Recovery." *JACS Journal, 4*(1), 2-3.

Gives and explains citations for Jewish prayers frequently used on JACS retreats.

412. (n.a.). (1986). "National Association of JACS Groups Formed." *JACS Journal, 3*(1), 1-2.

Describes the founding of JACS.

413. (n.a.). (1986). "National Conference on Addictions in the Jewish Community Marks Beginning." *JACS Journal, 3*(2), 1-2.

Reports on a conference concerning addiction in the Jewish community. Major recommendations from the conference are given.

414. O'Connell, T. (1989). "Jewish Alcoholics Face Unique Problems." *U.S. Journal of Drug and Alcohol Dependence, 13*(4), 8.

Describes some of the problems Jewish alcoholics encounter in AA and how JACS is helping them address those issues.

415. (n.a.). (1985). "Progress for Substance Abuse Education in Jewish Schools." *JACS Journal, 11*(1), 1-2.

Reports on the work being done by JACS to develop alcohol and other drug education programs.

416. Rabinowitz, R. (1986). "Alcoholism and Chemical Dependency in the Jewish Community: Sh...sh...sh." S. J. Levy & S. B. Blume (eds.), *Addiction in the Jewish Community.* (pp. 135-141). New York: Federation of Jewish Philanthropies of New York.

Explains the structure and purpose of JACS.

417. Richie, L. R. (27 April 1989). "Now There's A Help Group For Jewish Alcoholics." *Detroit Free Press*, 2B.

Describes JACS and gives references for Detroit area meetings.

418. Spiegel, M. C. (Summer, 1988). "Stigmatized Behavior: The Community Responds." *Genesis 2*, 21-22.

Describes the work that JACS and the L'Chaim Workshop is doing to help Jewish alcoholics.

419. Steinman, D. (1986). "A Jewish Spiritual Dictionary." *The JACS Journal*, *3*(2), 8-9.

Gives definitions of common terms used when discussing spirituality.

420. Vivian B. (1985). "A Fair Assessment." *The JACS Journal*, *2*(1), 2-3.

Member of JACS who staffed an information booth at the New York Self-Help Fair comments on denial.

421. Woolf, B. J. (1989). "Letter." *JACS Journal*, *6*(1), 7.

Compliments the work JACS does.

9

The Rabbi's Role in Recovery

422.   Aaron, M. (1990). "Rabbis Forum." *JACS Journal*, 7(1), 2.

Mentions limited training which Reform rabbis receive for dealing with addiction.

423.   (n.a.). (1982). "Alcoholism Among Jews: Special Interview with Abraham J. Twerski." *Alcoholism Update*, 5(4), 1,3.

Twerski explains cultural attitudes around alcoholism and what he considers to be a typical reaction an alcoholic Jew might encounter when talking to a rabbi.

424.   Almoni, P. (1986). "My Name Is Rabbi Almoni." *JACS Journal*, 3(1), 3, 9.

Tells of his addiction and recovery through AA. Special focus is placed on denial.

425.   American Business Men's Research Foundation. (6 August 1987). *Monday Morning Report*, 1-2.

Features a Gallup Poll report which "has indicated that the religious community in the U.S. is far from being actively involved in either ministry of healing or a ministry of prevention of alcohol problems."

426.   Anderson, G. W. (1982). "Candid Concern: The Church's Ministry to the Chemically Dependent Person (Alcoholism)." *Engage/ Social Action, 10*, 15-19.

Explains why ministers, priests, and rabbis have been ineffective in working with alcoholics. Suggests ways in which clergy can better minister to alcoholics.

427.   Birner, L. (1980). "The Rabbi and the Alcoholic Congregant." A. Blaine (ed.), *Alcoholism and the Jewish Community.* (pp. 311- 318). New York: Federation of Jewish Philanthropies of New York.

Describes how rabbis can identify alcohol problems, use intervention, and educate their congregations.

428.   Bloom, H. I. (1958). "Non-Alcoholics Need to Listen." *Box 1980, 15*(2), 26-28.

Describes the value of communication between alcoholics and non-alcoholics.

429.   Bloom, H. I. (1954). "A Rabbi Speaks." *Box 1980* [The Grapevine], *10*(10), 38-40.

Gives appraisal of AA from a Jewish perspective. Explains what rabbis can learn from attending open meetings.

430.   Blume, S. B., Dropkin, D., & Lokoliw, L. (1980). "The Jewish Alcoholic: A Descriptive Study." *Alcohol, Health and Research World, 4*(4), 21-26.

Reports on research with Jewish alcoholics. Lack of affiliation with the Jewish Community as a cause for alcoholism is addressed. Two alcoholic Orthodox rabbis studied.

431.   (n.a.). (1989). "Chaplaincy Training Program Becomes a Reality." *JACS Journal, 6*(1), 1,6.

Describes the chaplaincy training program developed by JACS to sensitize rabbis.

432.   Clinebell, H. J. (1966). *Basic Types of Pastoral Counseling.* New York: Abingdon Press.

Mention is made of rabbis who work with alcoholics.

433.   Clinebell, H. J. (1962). "Pastoral Care of the Alcohol's Family Before Sobriety." *Pastoral Psychology, 13,* 23+.

Pastoral ministers can help families decrease their fear and increase their supply of interpersonal satisfaction by "encouraging the family to re-establish social relationships--in the fellowship of the church and in Al-Anon."

434.   Clinebell, H. J. (1968). "Pastoral Counseling with the Alcoholic and His Family." In R. J. Catanzaro (ed.), *Alcoholism.* (pp. 189-207). Springfield: Charles C. Thomas.

Explaining why clergy are in a unique position to help alcoholics.

435.   Cohen, E. J. (1980). "AA at the International Synagogue, Kennedy Airport." A. Blaine (ed.), *Alcoholism and the Jewish Community.* (pp. 321-325). New York: Federation of Jewish Philanthropies of New York.

A personal account about how AA groups were established at the International Synagogue.

436.   Dulfano, C. (1977). "Stages of a Family Disease." *Sh'ma*,
        8(142), 191-192.

        Suggests that Jewish alcoholics get help from Rabbis.
        Focus is on how the family is affected by alcoholism.

437.   Einstein, S. (1970). "The Use and Misuse of Alcohol and
        Other Drugs." In G. Rosenthal (ed.), *The Jewish Family in
        a Changing World.* (pp. 86-121). Cranbury, NJ: Thomas
        Yoseloff.

        Reports on a survey of rabbis concerning the rate of
        alcoholism and other drug addiction in their congregations.

438.   Fenster, G. (1988). "Bottom Line Sobriety." *Alcoholism and
        Addiction, 8*(6), 6-7.

        Mentions a rabbi who argues that AA exposes many Jewish
        beliefs and that it is acceptable for Jews to say the Lord's
        Prayer at the close of AA meetings.

439.   Goodman, J. S. (1986). "The Knowledge of G-d's Will for
        the Price of a Phone Call." *JACS Journal, 3*(1), 4,12.

        Explains how the spirituality found in the twelve steps
        works in his life.

440.   Greisman, M. (21 March 1986). "Rabbi-Psychiatrist
        Concerned over Jewish Drug Problem." *Jewish Press*, 48.

        Mention is made of Rabbi Gringras, a recovered addict, and
        Rabbi Twerski, who works with alcoholics and other drug
        addicts.

441.   Gringras, Nd (n.d.). "Recovery and the Observant Jew."
        JACS Journal, 7(1), 6.

Argues that the joy of *Chassidus* or the spirit of *T'fila,
T'shuvah*, and *Tzedakah* serve as a basis for AA.

442. J. (1986). "Bill W. and the Rabbis." *The JACS Journal,
3*(2), 9.

Mentions reaction to a notice placed on the board at the
Central Conference of American Rabbis announcing a
hospitality suite for "Friends of Bill W."

443. (n.a.). (1984). "JACS Helps to Address Needs of Orthodox
Addicts." *JACS Journal, 1*(2), 1-2.

Reports on the successful efforts of JACS to help orthodox
Jewish men enter a treatment facility. Role of the
alcoholic's rabbi is addressed.

444. Kirschenbaum, S. S. (1987). "Substance Abuse: We are not
Immune." *Jewish News, 41*(10), 1, 24-25.

Reports on a conference on "Substance Abuse and Jews"
including the talk by Rabbi Nachem Gringras, a recovered
alcoholic and pill addict.

445. Koplowitz, I. (1923). *Midrash Yayin Veshechor: Talmudic
and Midrashic Exegetics on Wine and Strong Drink.*
Detroit: np.

"Presents the thoughts and sentiments of the Talmudic
Rabbis who were strongly opposed to the drinking of any
wine whatever." Written in Hebrew and English.

446. Kushner, P. (1980). "The Role of the Rabbi." A. Blaine
(ed.), *Alcoholism and the Jewish Community.* (pp. 305-309).
New York: Federation of Jewish Philanthropies of New
York.

Offers suggestions to rabbis who work with an alcoholic congregant.

447.   Levy, S. J. & Futernick, L. (1984). "Drinking and Drugging Among Jews." I. Trainin (ed.), *In the Path of Righteousness There is Life*. New York: Federation of Jewish Philanthropies.

Concentrates on the inability of many rabbis to recognize that alcoholics exist in their congregations.

448.   Levy, S. J. & Futernick, L. (1986). "Drinking and Drugging Among Jews." S. J. Levy & S. B. Blume (eds.), *Addictions in the Jewish Community*. (pp. 181-191). New York: Federation of Jewish Philanthropies of New York.

Originally appeared in Issac N. Trainin's (1984). *In the Path of Righteousness There is Life* New York: Federation of Jewish Philanthropies.

449.   Miller, Y. (1987). "Dear Rabbi." *JACS Journal*, 4(1), 4-5. How a rabbi can be a spiritual leader to Jewish alcoholics.

450.   (n.a.). (n.d.)."Rabbinical Seminaries Join to Develop Chaplaincy Curriculum on Substance Abuse." *JACS Journal*, 7(1), 1,7.

Describes educational programs being developed to train rabbis.

451.   Rice, O. R. (1944). "The Minister's Relation to the Alcoholic." In *Abridged Lectures of the First (1943) Summer Course on Alcohol Studies at Yale University*. (pp. 92-96). New Haven: Quarterly Journal of Studies on Alcohol.

Abridged version of Rice (1945) "Pastoral Counseling of Inebriates" *Alcohol, Science, and Society* New Haven: Quarterly Journal of Studies on Alcohol.

452. Rice, O. R. (1945). "Pastoral Counseling of Inebriates." In Anonymous (ed.), *Alcohol, Science, and Society.* (pp. 437-460). New Haven: Quarterly Journal of Studies on Alcohol.

Tells ways in which priests, ministers, and rabbis have a unique relationship with members of their congregations and how they can use the "tools of the trade" to assist in spiritual development. Limitations are also presented.

453. Rosenbloom, J.R. (January, 1964). "Alcoholism Addiction Among the Jews." *Central Conference of American Rabbis Journal, 11,* 56-61.

454. Simon, H. (1971). "The Jewish Community and the Use of Alcohol." *NCCA Blue Book, 23,* 105-109.

Emphasizes that Rabbis need to work to dispel the myth that there are no Jewish alcoholics. Mentions his own work in helping to establish the Shalom AA group.

455. Teller, B. (1989). "Chemical Dependency in the Jewish Community." *The Counselor, 7*(3), 27-28.

Describes need to sensitize rabbis and other professionals about the myth of Jewish immunity to alcoholism.

456. Trainin, I. (September/October 1977). "On Jewish Alcoholism." *Women's American ORT Reporter,* 9.

What rabbis can do to assist Jewish alcoholics.

457.   Trainin, I. (1987). "Interfaith Response to Alcoholism." *NCCA Blue Book*, *39*, 101-104.

        Argues for the creation of an inter-faith network to work with alcoholics.

458.   Trudeau, G. (March 12, 1989). "Doonesbury." *Detroit Free Press*, Comics section, p. 1.

        Punch line in this cartoon involves a rabbi walking into a bar.

459.   Twerski, A. J. (1981). "The Pastoral Counselor." In A. J. Twerski, *Caution: "Kindness" Can be Dangerous to the Alcoholic*. (pp. 92-98). Englewood Cliffs, NJ: Prentice-Hall.

        Uses a case study to demonstrate how a pastor can give faulty advice to an alcoholic and his wife.

460.   Twerski, A. J. (1984). "Understanding Alcoholism: A Personal Account." *JACS Journal*, *1*(2), 6-8.

        Tells how he became involved in the alcoholism field.

461.   Weiss, C. (6 February 1981). "Alcoholism Rises Among Jews." *Phoenix Jewish News*, 6-7.

        Focuses on the issue of denial, an issue which prevents rabbis from effectively working with alcoholics.

462.   Woolf, B. I. (1980). "A Personal Odyssey." A. Blaine (ed.), *Alcoholism and the Jewish Community*. (pp. 347-352). New York: Federation of Jewish Philanthropies of New York.

        Covers general issues concerning alcoholism in the Jewish Community.

463. Zimmermann, S. (1986). "Personal Reflections." S. J. Levy & S.B. Blume (eds.), *Addictions in the Jewish Community*. (pp. 87-90). New York: Federation of Jewish Philanthropies of New York.

Tells how author began working with Jewish alcoholics.

10

Alcoholism in Israel

464.   (n.a.). (week ending February 21, 1987). "Alcoholism on Rise." *Jerusalem Post*, International Edition.

The rise of alcohol related problems in Israel.

465.   Amer, M. & Eldar, P. (1978-1979). "An Experiment in the Treatment of Alcoholics in Israel." *Drug Forum*, 7(2), 105-119.

The myth that social and cultural traits exist which prevent Jews from becoming alcoholics. Reports on the rate of alcoholism in Israel.

466.   Antonovsky, H., Hankin, Y., & Stone, D. (1987). *British Journal of Addiction*, 82, 293.

Reports on research done of high risk Jews in Israel.

467.   Bar, C. & Bauml, R. (1982). *Habits of Consumption of Alcoholic Beverages Among the Israel Public*. Jerusalem: Israel Institute of Applied Research.

Reports on a survey they took to determine the attitudes and drinking behavior of the Jewish adult public.

468. Bar, H. & Bauml R. (1982). *Alcohol: Drinking Habits of the Jewish Public*. Jerusalem: Israel Institute of Applied Research.

Reports on the attitudes and behavior of the Israeli public.

469. Bar, H., Eldar, P., & Weiss, S. (1989). "Alcohol Drinking Habits and Attitudes of the Adult Jewish Population in Israel 1987." *Drug and Alcohol Dependence, 23*, 237-245.

"Present[s] attitudes towards alcohol drinking and non-ritual drinking habits in the general adult Jewish population in Israel." Found "a worrisome prevalence of non-ritual alcohol use."

470. Baras, M., Harlap, S., & Eisenberg, S. (1984). "Alcohol Drinking in Jerusalem." *Alcohol, 1*(6), 435-439.

Description of the rate of alcohol consumption in Jerusalem.

471. Bauml, R. & Eldar, P. (1983). "Drugs and Alcohol: Alcoholism in Israel." *Medicine and Law, 1*, 181-189.

Discusses problem of Jewish alcoholism in Israel which describes treatment and stresses the role of the family.

472. Ben-Yehuda, N. (1987). "Drug Abuse Social Policy in the United States and Israel: A Comparative Sociological Perspective." *International Journal of the Addictions, 22*(1), 17-45.

Concludes that while both the United States and Israel use the supply/demand reduction model to combat drug use, the program is more successful in Israel.

473. Ben-Yehuda, N. & Einstein, S. (1984). "Human Garbage and Physical Garbage: A Sociological Case Example of Institutional Violence." *International Journal of the Addictions, 19*(1), 1-23.

   Describes a methadone treatment program located in the largest garbage dump in Israel.

474. (n.a.). (1986). *Demographic Characteristics of Alcoholics in Treatment 1.4..85-31.3.86.* Jerusalem: Ministry of Labour and Social Affairs.

   Cited in Haviva Bar's "Alcohol Drinking Habits and Attitudes of the Adult Jewish Population in Israel, 1987" because it reports on Israeli treatment programs.

475. Einstein, S. (1979). "Drug Contagion in Jerusalem: A Pilot Investigation of the Israeli Drug Use Scene." *International Journal of the Addictions, 14*(3), 423-436.

   Interviewed 39 male and female adult Jewish and Arab street drug users in Jerusalem currently in treatment. "The most significant findings from this mini-study are that the majority of drug users did not initiate anyone else into drug use, and that those who did reported a variety of non-monetary gains."

476. Einstein, S. (1980). "Project Outreach: An Experimental Support System Intervention Program." *International Journal of the Addictions, 15*(1), 1-37.

   Describes a drug use intervention outreach program in Jerusalem.

477. Einstein, S. (1981). "Servicing the Drug User and the Drug User Treatment Support System." *International Journal of the Addictions, 16*(2), 185-196.

"Using a sample of male and female Israeli street polydrug users who were involved with a broad service support system, this paper analyzes and discusses the implications of meeting their multiple needs when delivery of care is the responsibility of specialized drug user treatment agencies."

478. Einstein, S. (1982). "Treating Drug Use and the Drug User: Factors and Issues to be Considered in the Development of a National Treatment Program." *International Journal of the Addictions, 17*(8), 1401-1417.

Describes the factors and issues which the author finds to be integral to the development of drug programs in Israel.

479. Eldar, P. (1977). "Alcoholism in Israel." *Public Health, 19,* 477-480.

480. Eldar, P. (1976). *An Israeli Experiment in the Treatment of Alcoholism.* Jerusalem: Department of International Relations.

Describes a two year experimental treatment program which involved treatment of the deprivation syndrome, treatment of drinking habits, and total abstinence from alcohol. Emphasis on vocational rehabilitation.

481. Eldar, P. (1983). *Residential Treatment Center for Alcoholics.* Jerusalem: Ministry of Labor and Social Affairs.

The objectives, treatment, and goals of residential treatment for alcoholics is explored in this report.

482. Eldar, P. & Yaffe, N. (1985). *Survey of Alcoholism in Israel in the First 25 Years Since the Establishment of the State.* Jerusalem, Israel: Ministry of Labor and Social Affairs.

Describes the history of alcohol use among Jews. No alcohol problem in Israel in the 1940s and 1950s, but the problem is increasing.

483.   Eldar, P. & Yaffe, N. (1986). "Survey of Alcoholism in Israel: The First Twenty-Five Years." S. J. Levy & S. B. Blume (eds.), *Addictions in the Jewish Community.* (pp. 103-121). New York: Federation of Jewish Philanthropies of New York.

Describes the growing rate of alcoholism in Israel. Treatment issues are discussed.

484.   Filman, M., Halpern, B., & Bauml, R. (1981). "L'alcoolisme en Israel." *L'Evolution Psychiatrique*, *46*(2), 461-471.

Found that alcohol is a growing problem in Israel. Describes a community based program of prevention and treatment. Text in French.

485.   Friedman, I. & Peer, I. (1968). "Drug Addiction Among Pimps and Prostitutes, Israel 1967." *International Journal of the Addictions*, *3*(2), 271-300.

Pimps and prostitutes begin using drugs after taking up delinquent activity. Prostitutes were not lured into prostitution through drugs.

486.   Harrison, J. (1978-79). "Some Characteristics of Young Israeli Drug Users." *Drug Forum*, *7*(2), 167-172.

Types of drugs used and reasons given for use by Israeli youth.

487. (n.a.). (May 8, 1981). "Hebrew Union College Communal Service Finds Alcohol Causing Problems for Israelis." *B'nai B'rith Messenger*, 9.

Reports on the problems of alcoholism and domestic violence in Israel.

488. Hes, J. P. (1970). "Drinking in a Yemenite Rural Settlement in Israel." *British Journal of Addictions*, *65*(4), 293-296.

"Presents information on drinking and drinking problems of a settlement located in the Jewish corridor and inhabited by Yemenite Jewish immigrants exclusively, except for two Moroccan families."

489. (n.a.). (n.d.). *Israel Society for the Prevention of Alcoholism.*

Handout which gives statistics about the rate of alcoholism in Israel.

490. Isralowitz, R. (1987). "Israel College Students' Drinking Problems: An Exploratory Study." *Psychological Reports*, *60*, 324-326.

Study of 156 Israeli college students suggested that while they drank less than American students, negative behavior is exhibited with use.

491. Javitz, R. & Shuvbal, J. T. (1982). "Vulnerability to Drugs Among Israeli Adolescents." *Israel Journal of Psychiatry*, *19*(2), 97-119.

Cited by Ben-Yehuda in "Drug Abuse Social Policy."

492. Joseph B. (October 29, 1986). "Move to Bar Drinks to Pupils." *Jerusalem Post*, 113.

This article is cited in Richard Isralowitz's "Kibbutz Youth and Alcohol Use."

493. Krasilowsky, D., Halpern, B., & Gutman, I. (1965). "The Problem of Alcoholism in Israel." *Israel Annals of Psychiatry and Related Disciplines*, *3*(2), 249-258.

   Research showed an increase in the production of alcohol, hospitalizations of alcoholic patients, and offenses committed under the influence of alcohol.

494. Lowenthal, U., Wald, D., & Klein, H. (1975). "Hospitalization of Alcoholics and the Therapeutic Community." *Harefuah*, *89*, 316- 320.

495. Mayer, R. R. "Drug Dependence in Israel." *Journal of Drug Issues*, *5*(1), 83.

496. Michaely, N., Eldar, P., & Weiss, S. (1989). *Journal of Substance Abuse Treatment*, *6*.

   Mentioned in Haviva Bar's "Alcohol Drinking Habits and Attitudes of the Adult Jewish Population in Israel, 1987" because it mentions treatment programs in Israel.

497. O'Connell, T. (1985). "Drinking and Drugging in the Holy Land" *Alcoholism: The National Magazine*, *5*(3), 22-23.

   Describes the growing use of alcohol among Jews in Israel.

498. Palgi, P. (1975). "The Traditional Role and Symbolism of Hashish Among Moroccan Jews in Israel and the Effect of Acculturation." V. Rubin (ed.), *Cannabis and Culture*. (pp. 207- 216). Mouton: The Hague.

   Why Israelis accept the use of Hashish by Moroccan Jews in Israel.

499. Richter, E., Metzer, U., Bloch, B., Tyger, G., & Ben-Dov, R. (1986). "Alcohol Levels in Drivers and Pedestrians Killed in Road Accidents in Israel." *International Journal of Epidemiology, 15*(2), 272-273.

Argues that "driving and walking while intoxicated...have emerged as public health problems in Israel." Comparisons are made between Jews, Moslems, and Christians.

500. Sagiv, M. (1979). "The Problem of Alcoholism in Israel." *Archives of Internal Medicine, 139*(3), 280-281.

Cites research that shows that the problem of alcoholism in Israel is growing.

501. Schachet, R. I. (1970). "The Rabbi and the Addict." G. Rosenthal (ed.), *The Jewish Family in a Changing World.* (pp. 136- 144). Cranbury, NJ: Thomas Yoseloff.

Explains some of the co-factors leading to drug abuse among Jewish youth.

502. Shoham, S. G., Geva, N., Kliger, D., & Chai, T. (1974). "Drug Abuse Among Israeli Youth: Epidemiological Pilot Study." *UN Bulletin of Narcotics, 26*(2), 9-28.

Purpose of study was to develop tools for a larger study. Some conclusions reported.

503. Shoham, S. G., Rahav, G., Esformer, V., Blau, J., Kaplinsky, N., Markovsky, R., & Woolf, B. (1978). "Differential Patterns of Drug Involvement Among Israeli Youth." *UN Bulletin on Narcotics, 30*(4), 17-34.

Describes the population of youth who are involved in drugs and compares them with those who are not.

504.   Shuval, R. & Krasilowsky, D. (1963). "A Study of Hospitalized Male Alcoholics." *Israel Annals of Psychiatry and Related Disciplines, 1*(2), 277-292.

Concludes that because "only 25 Jewish male alcoholics were found in Israel during 1961-1962" the problem of alcoholism is comparatively insignificant.

505.   Snyder, C. R., Palgi, P., Eldar, P., & Elian, B. (1982). "Alcoholism Among the Jews in Israel: A Pilot Study." *Quarterly Journal of Studies on Alcohol, 43*(7), 623-654.

Found that "there is a marked difference in the extent of alcoholism and related problems among Israeli Jews of the three major ethnic communities--Ashkenazi, Sephardic, and Oriental...--which may be explained sociologically in terms of historic differentiation of Jewish minorities from the drinking norms of surrounding majorities, liturgical differences prior to immigration, and differentials in the social stresses of post-immigration adaptation to life in modern Israel."

506.   Stolz, F. (1976). "Rausch, Religion, und Realitaet in Israel und Seiner Umwelt." *Vetus Testamentum, 26*, 170-186.

Discusses texts concerning the boundaries of sobriety in the realm of cult, wisdom, and prophecy in the ancient near east.

507.   Teichman, M., Rahav, G., & Barnea, Z. (1987). "Alcohol and Psychoactive Drug Use among Israeli Adolescents: An Epidemiological and Demographic Investigation." *International Journal of the Addictions, 22*(1), 81-92.

Describes moderate growth of substance abuse among Israeli adolescents.

508.   Van Dijk, M. (1984). "Recovery in the Promised Land"
        JACS Journal, 1(2), 11.

        Explains author's work as director of an alcoholism
        treatment center in Kiryat Gat, Israel.   Difficulty in
        beginning an AA group is discussed.

509.   Weiss, S. (1988). "Primary Prevention of Excessive
        Drinking and the Jewish Culture--Preventive Efforts in
        Israel 1984-1985." *Journal of Primary Prevention, 8*(4),
        218-225.

        For the people of Israel, responsible drinking can be
        accomplished by "changes in knowledge, attitudes,
        intentions and behavior."

510.   Weiss, S. (1985). *Teen-age Alcohol Consumption*:   *A
        Survey*. Jerusalem: Israeli Ministry of Labor and Social
        Affairs.

        Cited in Richard Isralowitz's "Kibbutz Youth and Alcohol
        Use."

511.   Wislicki, L. (1967). "Alcoholism and Drug Addiction in
        Israel." *British Journal of Addiction, 62*, 367-373.

        Marked increase in Israeli alcohol and hashish abuse over
        the past 20 years.

512.   Yaglom, M. & Krasilowsky, D. (1973). "The Problem of
        Drunkenness in Israel." *Harefua, 85*(2), 72-76.

11

Minorities within
the Jewish Community

WOMEN

513. Blume, S. (1982). "Psychiatric Problems of Alcoholic Women." In J. Solomon (ed.), *Alcoholism and Clinical Psychiatry.* (pp. 179-193). New York, New York: Plenum Medical Book Company.

Mentions Kant's 1798 observation that Jews and women avoid the appearance of drunkenness.

514. Blume, S. B. (July-August 1987). "Women's Health: Issues in Mental Health, Alcoholism, and Substance Abuse." *Public Health Reports Supplement,* 38-42.

Describes reasons why alcohol reacts differently in women than in men. Briefly mentions the historic belief that women, like Jews, have a low rate of alcoholism.

515. Blume, S. B. & D. Dropkin. (1980). "The Jewish Alcoholic Woman--Rara Avis?: General Characteristics and Particular Problems of Jewish Alcoholic Women." A. Blaine (ed.), *Alcoholism and the Jewish Community.* (pp. 275-293). New York: Federation of Jewish Philanthropies of New York.

Found that Jewish, alcoholic women were similar to other alcoholic women.

516. Corrigan, E. M. (1980). *Alcoholic Women in Treatment.* New York: Oxford University Press.

Classifies subjects as Catholic, Protestant, and other. Of the 14 women in the "other" category, 8 were Jewish.

517. Gringras, N. (February 1982). "Addiction Among Jewish People--What is Being Done?" *American Mizrachi Woman,* 16-17, 21.

Special attention is given to the disparity of attitudes toward male and female alcoholics.

518. Gringras, N. (February/March 1985). "Alcoholism and Addiction in the Jewish Community: A Progress Report." *Amit Women,* 18-20.

Describes the problem of alcoholism in the Jewish community, recovery through AA, how JACS can help Jews develop their spirituality in AA, and the need for Rabbis to be more involved in recovery.

519. Hornik, E.L. (1978). *The Drinking Woman.* New York: Associated Press.

Describes unique problems which Jewish, alcoholic women face in trying to recognize their addiction and to get treated for it.

520. Hornik, E.L. (1978). "The Drinking Jewish Woman." *Jewish Digest,* 26(3), 36-40.

Extracted from her book *The Drinking Woman,* New York: Associated Press.

521.   Lois R. (1989). "Jewish Alcoholics." *The Journal, 13*(5), 4.

Writes that as a Jewish alcoholic, she was stigmatized as both a Jew and a woman.

522.   Mello, N. K. (1980). "Some Behavioral and Biological Aspects of Alcohol Problems in Women." In O. J. Kalant (ed.), *Alcohol and Drug Problems in Women: Research Advances in Alcohol and Drug Problems*. Volume 5. (pp. 263-298). New York, New York: Plenum Press.

Brief mention is made of the low incidence of alcoholism among Jews.

523.   Schneider, S. W. (1984). *Jewish and Female: Choices and Changes in Our Lives Today*. New York: Simon and Schuster.

Claims that Jewish women feel more alienated from their religion than do men. As a result, it is more difficult for them to tap into their heritage while in recovery. Case studies cited.

524.   Spiegel, M. C. (1986). "Alcoholism: Jewish Women Confront a Growing Problem." S. J. Levy & S. B. Blume (eds.), *Addictions in the Jewish Community*. (pp. 62-74). New York: Federation of Jewish Philanthropies of New York.

Explains issues facing alcoholic, Jewish women. AA is mentioned throughout.

525.   Thompson, K. M. & Wilsnack, R. W. (1984). "Drinking and Drinking Problems Among Female Adolescents: Patterns and Influences." S. C. Wilsnack & L. J. Beckman (eds.), *Alcohol Problems in Women*. (pp. 37-65). New York: Guilford Press.

Argues that "those [adolescents] with Irish backgrounds were more likely to drink, get drunk, and report drinking problems than adolescents with Italian, English or Jewish backgrounds."

526.   (February/March 1985). "Turning Point." *Amit Women*, 19.

Jewish woman tells about her addiction and recovery with the help of JACS.

527.   Weiss, C. (20 February 1988). "Two Valley Women Win Battle with Bottle." *Phoenix Jewish News, 8*, 8-9.

Case studies of two female, Jewish alcoholics who recovered through AA.

528.   (1979). "Woman Alcoholic Shares Her Struggle." *NCA News: From the Alcoholism Council of the South Bay, 2*(1), 1,3.

Brief story by a Jewish woman who is an alcoholic.

YOUTH

529.   (n.a.). (December 1981). "Addiction Self-Help Formed for Orthodox Jews." *Young Israel Viewpoint.*

Description of a special interest AA meeting formed for Orthodox Jews.

530.   Adler, I. & Kandel, D. B. (1981). "Cross Cultural Perspectives on Developmental Stages in Adolescent Drug Abuse." *Journal of Studies on Alcohol, 42*(9), 701-715.

Compared French and Israeli students. Found cumulative sequence of alcohol and drug use.

531. Birner, L. (1973). "Adolescent Suicide." L. Landman (ed.), *Judaism and Drugs*. (pp. 165-171). New York: Federation of Jewish Philanthropies of New York.

      Argues that the drug culture combines adolescent death games (such as "chicken") with adult quests for money.

532. Davids, L. (1982). "Ethnic Identity, Religiosity, and Youthful Deviance: The Toronto Computer Dating Project--1979." *Adolescence*, *17*(67), 673-684.

      Measured how religiosity and ethnic identity affected the drug use and premarital sexual activity of Jewish youth.

533. Dinai, A. & Lerner, M. (1981). "The Single Drug User and His Audience." *International Journal of the Addictions*, *16*(6), 1003- 1008.

      Describes hashish and pep pill usage by a single individual in a group context. Advice on intervention techniques which can be used to work with such an individual.

534. Fishman, R. (1980). "Drinking Among Teenagers." A. Blaine (ed.), *Alcoholism and the Jewish Community*. (pp. 255-273). New York: Federation of Jewish Philanthropies of New York.

      Discusses rates of alcoholism and alcohol abuse among youth.

535. Flanzer, J. P. (1979). "Alcohol Use Among Jewish Adolescents: A 1977 Sample." In M. Galanter (ed.), *Currents in Alcoholism*. (pp. 257-268). New York, New York: Grune and Stratton.

Surveyed Jewish high school students. Findings support Snyder's in-group/out-group hypothesis and Bales 1964 analysis delimiting drinking behaviors.

536. Flanzer, J. P. (1980). "Alcohol Use Among Jewish Adolescents." A. Blaine (ed.), *Alcoholism and the Jewish Community*. (pp. 135- 151). New York: Federation of Jewish Philanthropies of New York.

Found that Jewish youth's use of alcohol and other drugs was comparable to the general increase of drug use among youth.

537. Friedman, M. I. (1973). "The Counter-Force Program." L. Landman (ed.), *Judaism and Drugs*. (pp. 245-257). New York: Federation of Jewish Philanthropies of New York.

Describes the Counter-Force Program of Torah Umasorah which was designed to help prevent Jewish youth from using drugs. A case study shows how this program works.

538. Frimer, N. E. (1973). "Jewish Students and Drugs on the Campus." L. Landman (ed.), *Judaism and Drugs*. (pp. 147-164). New York: Federation of Jewish Philanthropies of New York.

Describes how Jewish students are being affected by drug use on college campuses.

539. Goldsmith, E.H., Laibson, A.S., Kaplan, & others. (April, 1986). "Teenage Life: How Do I Deal with Substance Abuse?" *Keeping Posted, 31,* 5.

540. Isralowitz, R. & Anson, J. (1988). "Kibbutz Youth and Alcohol Use: Patterns and Problems." *Journal of Alcohol and Drug Education, 34*(1), 60-63.

Concludes that Kibbutz youth use alcohol no less than other Israeli youth.

541.   Jackson, B. (1975). "Psychology, Psychiatry, and the Pastor: Part IV, the Spiritual Dimension of Drug Abuse." *Bibliotheca Sacra, 132*, 291-303.

Argues that to halt drug abuse, youth must be introduced to Jesus Christ. Section on historical issues mentions the Talmud and traditional Jewish interpretation of selected passages.

542.   Kaufman, E. & Borders, L. (1984). "Adolescent Substance Abuse in Anglo-American Families." *Journal of Drug Issues, 14*(2), 365-377.

Examines healthy Anglo-American families to identify characteristics of the family systems which help "prevent adolescent substance abuse even in the face of heavy peer pressure."

543.   Kraut, B. (1973). "Perspectives on the Drug Issue." L. Landman (ed.), *Judaism and Drugs*. (pp. 187-222). New York: Federation of Jewish Philanthropies of New York.

Addresses student attitudes toward marijuana use and a general analysis of the drug problem before proposing a proper Jewish response to marijuana use.

544.   Landman, R. (1952). "Studies of Drinking in Jewish Culture III: Drinking Patterns of Children and Adolescents Attending Religious Schools." *Quarterly Journal of Studies on Alcohol, 13*(1), 87-94.

Studied Jewish youth ages 5-17 who attended Jewish schools in New Haven, CT. Concludes that this generation of Jews will show a high incidence of drinking with a low incidence of excessive drinking.

545.   Leffler, W. J. "Middle Class Jewish Youth and Drug Abuse." *Journal of Drug Issues, 3*(4), 318.

546.   Levinson, R. D. (16 September 1971). "Drugs Ravage Jewish Youth." *The Jewish Chronicle*, 7.

Cited by Norman Frimer in "Jewish Students and Drugs." There are several newspapers published under the title *Jewish Chronicle*. We have been unable to identify which newspaper includes this article.

547.   McCarthy, R. G. (1959). "High School Drinking Studies." In R. G. McCarthy (ed.), *Drinking and Intoxication*. (pp. 205-210). New Haven: Yale Center of Alcohol Studies.

Religious affiliation is used as one of the variables studied.

548.   McGonegal, J. (1972). "The Role of Sanction in Drinking Behavior." *Quarterly Journal of Studies on Alcohol, 33*(3a), 692-697.

Investigates parental attitudes/actions toward alcohol use and the affects of these actions/attitudes on their children's alcohol use. Religious sanction is stressed.

549.   (n.a.). (1983). *Overview and Key Findings*. Charlotte, NC: Charlotte Drug Education Center.

Study of high school students in which Jews were the second highest group of drug users.

550.   Pearlman, S., Phillip, A. F., & Robbins, L. C. (1972). "Religious Affiliations and Patterns of Drug Usages in an Urban University Population." *Proceedings of First*

International Conference on Student Drug Surveys. Farmingdale: Baywood Publishing.

551. (n.a.). (1980). *Religiosity and Drug Use: A Study of Jewish and Gentile College Students.* Rockville: Alcohol, Drug Abuse, and Mental Health Administration.

552. Rosenthal, M. S. (1986). "Youthful Drug Abuse and the Jewish Family." S. J. Levy & S. B. Blume (eds.), *Addictions in the Jewish Community.* (pp. 145-159). New York: Federation of Jewish Philanthropies of New York.

General discussion of alcoholism and other drug addiction among youth.

553. Schrage, S. (1973). "A Hassidic Approach to Alienated Youth." L. Landman (ed.), *Judaism and Drugs.* (pp. 173-186). New York: Federation of Jewish Philanthropies of New York.

Argues that the Jewish community should develop anti-drug programs "that stress Jewish identity, philosophy and ethics" instead of duplicating existing programs.

554. Shoham, S. G., Rahav, G., Esformes, Y., Blau, J., Kaplinsky, N., Markovsky, R., & Woolf, B. (1981). "Polar Types of Reported Drug Involvement Among Israeli Youth." *International Journal of the Addictions, 16*(7), 1161-1167.

Focused on the marijuana use of 776 boys and girls (aged 14-18) in an attempt to identify and describe types of youth drug involvement.

555. Shoham, S. G., Rahav, G., Esformes, Y., Chard, F., & Kaplinsky, N. (1980). "Some Parameters of the Use of Alcohol by Israeli Youth and Its Relationship to Their

Involvement with Cannabis and Tobacco." *Drug and Alcohol Dependence, 6,* 263-272.

Higher alcohol consumption is associated with youth with a profile of delinquency, personal problems, or low parental control.

556. Spiegel, M. C. (1977). "Is Alcoholism the New Jewish Disease?" *Sh'ma, 8*(142), 189-191.

Argues that when Jewish youth retain traditional customs regarding drinking, alcoholism was greatly decreased.

557. Straus, R. & Bacon, S. D. (1953). *Drinking in College.* New Haven: Yale University Press.

Study of college drinking which includes disproportionately large number of Jews and Mormons.

LESBIANS AND GAY MEN

558. (n.a.). (1988). "Holiday Highlights." *Our Voice, 3*(2), 3.

Mention is made that Pride Institute displayed a menorah and that Jewish patients conducted a daily ceremony as a celebration of Chanukah.

559. (n.a.). (1989). "Holiday Highlights at Pride." *Our Voice, 4*(3), 4.

Efforts at Pride Institute to accommodate the spiritual beliefs of their clients. Special meals and events commemorate Chanukah, Christmas, and the Solstice.

560. Lewis. (1990). "Abusive Childhoods." (pp. 273-295) *Circle of Hope.* P. Tilleraas (ed). Center City, MN: Hazelden.

Shares childhood experiences of growing up in an alcoholic family as well as personal experiences with alcoholism and other drug addictions, recovery through AA, and diagnosis with AIDS. Maternal grandparents were Russian Jews.

561. (n.a.). (1982). "Liberated Woman." *The Way Back.* 1981. (pp. 65-74). Washington, D.C.: Whitman-Walker Clinic.

Jewish woman tells about her period of liberation--as a lesbian and as a woman--after joining AA.

562. McNally, E. B. (1989). *Lesbian Recovering Alcoholics in Alcoholics Anonymous: A Qualitative Study of Identity Transformation.* New York University, New York.

Studies experiences of eight lesbian alcoholics to determine how they integrated their lesbian and alcoholic identities. Two of the women came from Jewish households.

563. (n.a.). (1989). "Workshops at Pride: Lesbians and Chemical Dependency." *Our Voice, 4*(3), 1.

Workshop on "Lesbian Minorities" included information on Jewish lesbians.

BLACKS

564. Singer, M. (1980). "The Function of Sobriety Among Black Hebrews." *Journal of Operational Psychiatry, 11*(2), 162-168.

Argues that among black Hebrews in Israel "institutionalized sobriety functions to promote anxiety-maintenance" and that "anxiety is deliberately fostered...as an adaptive response to internal and external threat."

12

Literary Portrayals

565.   Begg, C. (1980). "Bread, Wine, and Strong Drink in Deut 29: 5A." *Bijdragen Tijdschrift Voor Filosophie En Theology, 41,* 266- 275.

Cites several Old Testament texts in relation to Deuteronomy 29:5 and concludes that Yahweh denied the Israelis these beverages so that their religious perceptions that Yahweh is Lord would not be obscured.

566.   Bellow, S. *The Victim.* New York: Vanguard Press, 1947.

567.   Berryman, J. (1975). *Recovery.* New York: Farrar, Straus, and Giroux.

Describes addiction, attempted recovery, and AA. As with his poetry, religion takes a central role in the novel.

568.   Bloom, H. I. (1951). "Twelfth Step." *Box 1980* [The Grapevine], *8*(5), 24-25.

Interprets the AA program in a poem.

569.   Elbert, J. (1980). *Murder at A.A.* New York, New York: NAL Penguin Inc.

A minor character is a Chinese-American alcoholic who converted to Judaism.

570. Forseth, R. (1985). "'Alcoholite at the Altar': Sinclair Lewis, Drink, and the Literary Imagination." *Modern Fiction Studies, 31*(3), 581-607.

   Analysis of Sinclair Lewis' writing. Jews are cited as having a low rate of alcoholism.

571. Gilmore, T. B. (1987). *Equivocal Spirits: Alcoholism and Drinking in Twentieth-Century Literature*. Chapel Hill: University of North Carolina Press.

   One chapter discusses Saul Bellow's *The Victim*.

572. Goldberg, D. [trans.] (n.d.). *Mashkeh*. Brooklyn, New York: Operation Survival.

   Translates Jewish teachings on alcohol use. The text is in both English and Hebrew.

573. Goodenough, E. R. (1958). *Jewish Symbols of the Greco-Roman Period*. New York: Pantheon.

   Volumes 5 and 6 focus on wine use. Topics include wine in Jewish archeology, ritualistic drinking, and wine in literary expression.

574. Goodwin, D. W. (1970). "The Alcoholism of F. Scott Fitzgerald." *Journal of the American Medical Association, 212*(1), 86-90.

   Argues that "alcoholism is unevenly distributed among groups. More men than women are alcoholic, more Irishmen than Jews, more bartenders than bishops."

575.   Jellinek, E. M. (1941). "Immanuel Kant on Drinking."
       Quarterly Journal of Studies on Alcohol, 1(4), 777-778.

       Comments that Kant found that alcoholism was rare among
       Jews.

576.   Jong, E. (1990). *Any Woman's Blues*. New York: Harper
       and Row.

       Main character is an alcoholic, sexually addicted Jewish
       artist.

577.   Leskov, N. S. (1957). "Nesmertel'nyi Golovan" [Deathless
       Golovan]. *Complete   Works.   6   1880;   Moscow:*
       Gos-izd-khudozh.

578.   McKinlay, A. P. (1948). "Ancient Experience with
       Intoxicating Drinks: Non-Classical Peoples." *Quarterly
       Journal of Studies on Alcohol, 9*(3), 387-414.

       Describes reactions of both secular and religious Jewish
       writers to use of wine.

579.   McKinlay, A. P. (1959). "Non-Classical Peoples." R. G.
       McCarthy (ed.), *Drinking and Intoxication.* (pp. 62-72).
       New Haven, CT: College and University Press.

       Includes information on Jewish experience with wine. The
       article is taken form his "Ancient Experience with
       Intoxicating Drinks" which appeared in (1948) *Quarterly
       Journal of Studies on Alcohol, 9*, 388-414.

580.   Patai, R. (1980). "From 'Journey Into the Jewish Mind'--
       Alcoholism." A. Blaine (ed.), *Alcoholism and the Jewish
       Community.* (pp. 61-87). New York: Federation of Jewish
       Philanthropies of New York.

Investigates mythical, moralistic, and laudatory references to wine found in the Bible and the Talmud.

581. Rubin, M. (1987). *The Boiled Frog Syndrome*. Boston: Alyson Publications, Inc.

The low incidence of alcoholism in the Jewish Community and the fact that "Shickuv vi a goy" is important to one of the subplots in this novel about the resistance movement against the theocracy which took control of the United States.

582. Taintor, E. ([pseud.]). (1945). *September Remember*. New York: Prentice Hall.

A novel of addiction and recovery through AA in which the comment is made that Jews cannot become "rum hounds."

583. Tendler, M. D. (1973). "Ethical Implications of the Drug Culture." L. Landman (ed.), *Judaism and Drugs*. (pp. 61-69). New York: Federation of Jewish Philanthropies of New York.

Explains what Torah ethics has to say abut the drug scene.

Author Index

Title Index

Subject Index

About the Compiler

STEVEN L. BERG is a consultant in the field of alcoholism and drug abuse. He has written at length about substance abuse and spiritual issues. His most recent book is *Alcoholism and Recovery: A Manual for the Pastoral Ministry* (1989).

www.ingramcontent.com/pod-product-compliance
Lightning Source LLC
Chambersburg PA
CBHW050228270326
41914CB00003BA/622

* 9 7 8 0 3 1 3 2 7 6 0 3 3 *